OXFORD MEDICAL PUBLICATI

Health for All Children

This book is

Health for All Children

Report of the Third Joint Working Party on Child
Health Surveillance

THIRD EDITION

Edited by

DAVID M. B. HALL

Professor of Community Paediatrics,
University of Sheffield,
Children's Hospital, Sheffield

Oxford   New York   Tokyo
OXFORD UNIVERSITY PRESS

Oxford University Press, Walton Street, Oxford OX2 6DP

Oxford   New York

Athens   Auckland   Bangkok   Bombay
Calcutta   Cape Town   Dar es Salaam   Delhi
Florence   Hong Kong   Istanbul   Karachi
Kuala Lumpur   Madras   Madrid   Melbourne
Mexico City   Nairobi   Paris   Singapore
Taipei   Tokyo   Toronto

and associated companies in
Berlin   Ibadan

Oxford is a trade mark of Oxford University Press

Published in the United States
by Oxford University Press Inc., New York

First edition 1989
Second edition 1991
Third edition 1996
Reprinted 1996
Reprinted 1996 (with corrections)

A catalogue record for this book is available from the British Library

Library of Congress Cataloging in Publication Data
(Data available)
ISBN 0 19262656 6

Typeset by Footnote Graphics, Warminster, Wilts
Printed in Great Britain by
Bookcraft Ltd, Midsomer Norton, Avon

Foreword to the third edition

Professor Sir Michael Peckham
Director of Research and Development, Department of Health

The first two editions of *Health for all children* looked at the content of Child Health surveillance and emphasized the importance of applying rigorous criteria for screening programmes in community child health. In particular, the role and value of screening for hearing loss, vision defects, hip dislocation, and a range of other conditions were discussed. The recommendations achieved their desired effect and the results of research relevant to this important area are described in the third edition. The reports raise new questions but it is gratifying that the prevention of ill health in children is now firmly on the research agenda.

This new edition considers child health promotion, by which is meant the primary prevention of childhood ill health. The various goals and the means by which they may be achieved are discussed in detail. Although randomized controlled trials can play a valuable role in this field, they are difficult to design and execute. It will be some years before it will be possible to say with confidence what does or does not work, for whom, and in what circumstances.

Health service providers and commissioners, like managers in many other fields, are obliged to make decisions which are often not supported by sound research evidence. Given the gaps in our knowledge it is important that research is sustained at a sufficient level to enable effective new approaches to the prevention of ill health in children to be devised.

The immediate challenge is four-fold: to define more precisely the aims of preventive child health services at local level; to ensure that preventive interventions relevant to those aims are soundly based; to devise better methods of allocating and deploying existing resources; and to ensure that there is an effective mechanism for evaluating the impact of child health promotion more reliably.

Introduction to the third edition

The surveillance and monitoring of child health, growth, and development are regarded as good practice throughout the Western world. Until the mid-1980s it was assumed that the value of these activities was self-evident, but there was then, and still is now, a striking paucity of research into the individual tests and other components of the various surveillance programmes. Over the past decade there has been an increasingly critical approach to all forms of surveillance and screening. Limitations in resources and demands for a rational approach to resource allocation have made it essential to evaluate health care activities and seek the most cost-effective means of delivery.

Surveillance, like other aspects of health care, has to be sensitive to the views of the consumer. Parents expect to be consulted about and participate in decisions that involve their children, and increasingly are prepared to challenge professional expertise and advice. The introduction of the parent-held record, the patients' charter, and the United Nations Convention on the Rights of the Child[1] are a response to this changing climate of opinion. The radical disability rights movement has rejected the 'labelling' of individuals and stressed the role of society in creating handicap.[2] Similarly, in the field of special education there has been a move away from diagnostic labelling or categorization, and more emphasis is placed on a descriptive analysis of each child's strengths and weaknesses. These changing ideas must be reflected in the ways in which health professionals define their aims and their methods of assessment and intervention.

Despite the impetus to research created by these pressures, there are still many gaps in our knowledge about the effectiveness of preventive child health activities. There are wide variations in the pattern of preventive child health services between countries, and these cannot be attributed solely to differing socio-economic conditions.[3] Even within the UK, until 1989 (when the first edition of *Health for all children* was published), there was no uniformity regarding either the number or the content of developmental surveillance examinations. Many health authorities were unable either to specify the precise nature of their programme or to produce evidence of its effectiveness.[4] Individual clinicians rightly felt that they had a duty to provide what they regarded as optimal care in the light of local conditions.[5] Nevertheless, it was possible to establish a core programme based on considerations of validity and efficiency which was considered acceptable by most health professionals throughout the UK.[6]

There have been many changes in health care since the first edition,[7] including* the reorganization of the NHS (NHS and Community Care Act 1990), the Children Act 1989, the New Contract for General Practice 1990, the Education Reform Act 1988, and the Education Act 1993 (including Code of Practice 1994). Much of routine child health surveillance has now moved into general practice and attendance at community clinics has declined. Community doctors spend less time in surveillance and more in specialist consultation and problem solving. The role of the health visitor as the key point of professional contact for parents is perhaps more important than ever before.[8]

Nevertheless, much remains to be done. Despite the extensive debate surrounding the publication of *Health for all children* and the apparent broad measure of consensus achieved, there are still wide variations in policies, priorities, and standards between districts. Many districts have as yet failed to specify their aims, procedures, referral criteria, or referral routes. Arrangements for the monitoring and audit of child health surveillance, and the integration of child health services, are still unsatisfactory in many districts.

How the review was done

Child health promotion and surveillance incorporate a wide variety of activities and it would be futile to consider such a complex programme as a single entity. The first Joint Working Party decided that the only way to proceed was to list the various aims identified by child health professionals and the means by which they might be achieved. Each component could then be analysed in detail.

We followed the same approach for this third edition. We attempted to synthesize the available evidence from a variety of disciplines, including medicine and nursing, the therapy professions, psychology, education, and social sciences. Particular weight was given to randomized controlled trials, but they are few in number in the areas surveyed. Many other types of study design have also been considered. We have

* For the equivalent legislation in Scotland, see p. xii.

kept in mind the hazards of selective literature reviews and incomplete searches, though in view of the breadth of the topic it is inevitable that some studies will have been overlooked[9]. We compiled our bibliography with the help of experts who have themselves carried out recent reviews and hope that as a result we have not omitted many major contributions to the literature.

The review included the following.

1. Studies on the individual elements of health care: for example, a specific examination such as the neonatal review, a procedure such as testing hearing, or a programme with a clearly identified aim such as reducing the number of scalds caused by hot bath water.
2. Reports on projects with a range of aims and outcome measures, such as a health visiting project designed for a specific sector of the population.
3. Reports on community projects such as Newpin.
4. Reflective and philosophical articles, anecdotal reports, and reviews of professional opinion and practice.
5. Work on the general principles of health care: for example, the criteria for screening programmes or the role of health economic analyses.

Future editions

The Joint Working Party hopes that this new edition will be a stimulus and a guide for all who are interested in preventive care and health promotion for children. We are aware, as we were with the previous two editions, that new research may invalidate much of what is written here. Our recommendations are in our view 'today's best buy'. They must be kept under constant scrutiny and we hope that as a result of new research stimulated by *Health for all children*, they will need to be updated within a few years.

Notes and references

1. Children's Rights Development Unit (1994). *UK agenda for children.* CRDU, London.
2. Coleridge, P. (1993). *Disability, liberation and development.* Oxfam Publications, Oxford.
3. Anonymous (1990). Child health in 1990: the United States compared to

Canada, England and Wales, France, The Netherlands, and Norway. Proceedings of a Conference, Washington, DC, 18–19 March 1990. *Pediatrics* 86, 1025–1127.
4. Butler, J. (1989). *Child health surveillance in primary care: a critical review*. HMSO, London.
5. Elfer, P. and Gatiss, S. (1990). *Charting child health services*. National Children's Bureau, London.
6. Jones, A. and Bilton, K. (1994). *The future shape of children's services*. National Children's Bureau, London.
7. Butler, J., Freidenfeld, K., and Relton J. (1995). *Child health surveillance in the new NHS*. Report to the Department of Health, University of Kent, (Centre for Health Services Studies).
8. Gillam, S., Glickman, M., Boyle, G., and Woodroffe, C. (1993). Cooperation or conflict over Child Health Surveillance? Views of key actors. *Quality in Health Care* 2, 83–6.
9. Chalmers I. and Altman D.G. (1995). *Systematic reviews*. BMJ, London.

Acknowledgements

The members of the Working Party, and the Editor in particular, are immensely grateful to all those who have assisted with the preparation of this third edition. Some have read and commented on sections of the manuscript or, in some cases, the whole of it; others have provided references, unpublished literature reviews, books, or suggestions based on experience or local audits.

To thank every individual and organisation by name here would require several pages and would risk omitting one or more of our contributors. Furthermore, we have not been able to use or adopt every suggestion made to us and are aware that some colleagues may not agree with our conclusions. We hope, therefore, that you will accept our thanks and forgive us for not listing you here. Wherever possible, due acknowledgment has been made by quoting the appropriate reference or bibliography.

A Note on the bibliography

The first two editions of *Health for all children* contained a substantial bibliography, comprising some 500 references and 35 pages. In compiling the third edition, over 2000 articles, books and other publications were considered, either by the members of the Working Party or by those providing advice and opinions. Inclusion of all these references would have greatly increased the size and price of the book.

We have therefore provided only a brief bibliography at the end of each chapter. For those who seek a more substantial list of sources for further private study, a separate bibliography is available. This can be provided either on disk or on paper. For further details, please contact:

The British Paediatric Association
5, St Andrew's Place
Regents Park
London NW1 4LB
Tel: 0171 486 6151
Fax: 0171 486 6009

Acknowledgements

Many people sent us articles and other publications. The following made substantial contributions to the bibliography within their particular areas of expertise:

Jennifer Gallagher and Jane Goodman (dental disease); Carol Dezateux and Ian Leck (hip disorders); Down's Syndrome Association (Jennifer Dennis); HemoCue Ltd (iron deficiency); Posey Marriage (effects of hearing loss); James Law and Pam Enderby (speech and language); Kate Saffin (Personal Child Health Records).

I am grateful to Jenny Milner and Eric Holroyd who gave vital assistance with managing the references database.

Dr Mitch Blair provided much of the material for Chapter 13.

Note for readers in Scotland

Certain references to legislation, etc., made in the text are not relevant to Scotland. References to districts includes health boards. For the most part the Children Act does not apply and the equivalent, when enacted, will be The Children (Scotland) Bill. The relevant Education Act is the Education (Scotland) Act 1980. The equivalent of *Health of the Nation* is *Scotland's Health: A Challenge to Us All*.

Note for readers in Wales

The health gain document is *Protocol for investment in health gain*, Welsh Office, NHS, and Welsh Health Planning Forum, 1991.

Contents

Overview of the 1995 programme   1

Clearer pre-school focus   1
New terminology   1
How will the changes affect the Primary Health Care Team and
  the General Practitioner?   1
Workload and resource implications   2
CHP tasks, services, and goals   2
Needs assessment and targeting   3
A health services partnership   3
Partnership with other agencies   3
Improvements in CHS   3
Physical examination   4
Regular CHS reviews   4
Growth monitoring   5
Hearing screening   5
Vision screening   5
Laboratory and radiological procedures   5
Iron deficiency   5
Developmental reviews   5
Child mental health   6
Information systems   6
Personal child health records   6

1 Health for all children   7

Definitions and concepts   10
The need for an evidence-based child health service   16
Recommendations   17
Notes and references   18

2 Child health promotion   19

Whose responsibility?   20
The tasks of health promotion   21

Ethical considerations   27
Problems in the evaluation of CHP   28
Evidence of effectiveness—lessons from the literature review   30
Implications for CHP—targeting and its problems   33
Recommendations—the key aims   36
Notes and references   38

3 Opportunities for primary prevention   41

Reducing the incidence of infectious diseases   41
Prevention of sudden infant death syndrome and sudden
   unexpected death in infancy   44
Reduction of smoking by parents   44
Prevention of unintentional injury   45
Nutrition   51
Dental and oral disease   54
Special situations   57
Recommendations   57
Notes and references   58

4 Promoting child development   61

Aims   61
'Good enough' parenting skills   61
The relationship between mothers' mental health and child
   development   63
Promoting language acquisition—looking ahead to school   65
Primary prevention of behavioural and psychological
   problems   67
Child protection—prevention of child abuse and neglect   68
What evidence of effectiveness is available?   70
Conclusion   73
Recommendations   74
Notes and references   74

**5 Secondary prevention: early detection and the role of
   screening**   77

Does early detection matter?   77
How early detection is achieved   79
All parents need help sometimes—the role of professional
   advice   81

The role of formal screening programmes   82
The need for professional sensitivity   82
Screening   82
Notes and references   89

6 **Physical examination**   90

Neonatal and 8-week examinations   90
School entrant medical examination   91
Individual physical examination procedures   92
Recommendations   103
Notes and references   107

7 **Growth monitoring**   109

Value of growth monitoring   109
Benefits of growth monitoring   110
Weight monitoring   112
Length and height monitoring   114
Requirements for successful growth monitoring   116
Recommendations for growth monitoring   121
Head circumference   125
Appendix: Regression to the mean   127
Notes and references   129

8 **Laboratory and radiological screening tests**   130

Neonatal phenylketonuria and congenital hypothyroidism   130
Other inherited metabolic disorders   132
Cystic fibrosis   132
Muscular dystrophy   133
Urine infections   133
Screening for haemoglobinopathies   134
Liver disease in infancy: extrahepatic biliary atresia   135
Familial hypercholesterolaemia   135
Atlanto-axial instability in people with Down's syndrome   136
Subclinical lead poisoning   136
Other screening programmes   136
Recommendations   137
Notes and references   139

9 Iron deficiency   140

Definition   140
Effects   140
Prevalence   141
Screening   141
Primary prevention   142
Recommendations   144
Notes and references   145

10 Screening for hearing defects   146

The nature of hearing impairment   146
Early diagnosis and intervention   149
Recommendations   158
Notes and references   162

11 Screening for vision defects   164

Conditions causing a disabling vision impairment as the
   primary problem   164
Screening for common non-incapacitating vision defects   165
Is there a case for preschool screening for vision defects?   170
School entrant screening   171
Detection of squints   171
Community screening—evidence and options   171
Colour vision defects   173
Vision and 'dyslexia'   173
Recommendations   174
Notes and references   177

12 Disorders of development and behaviour   179

Disability   179
Low-prevalence high-severity conditions   180
High-prevalence low-severity conditions   184
Problems with applying the concept of screening to
   development and behaviour   199
Routine developmental assessments for all school entrants?   203
Measuring the effectiveness of routine developmental
   screening and assessment   204

A pragmatic approach—reconciling varying views by setting
    agreed priorities   204
Recommendations   207
Notes and references   209

13 Organization, management, and records   212

Introduction   212
The tasks involved in a successful CHP programme   213
Data collection   215
Quality checklist   216
Litigation   218
Personal child health records   219
Notes and references   221

14 Summary of 1995 child health promotion programme   223

Introduction   223
The core surveillance programme for individual children   225

Appendix 1   233
Appendix 2   234
Index   237

An Overview of the 1996 Programme

How does this edition of *Health for all children* differ from the last two? This chapter summarizes the main changes and the most important elements of the 1996 programme for child health.

Clearer pre-school focus

Although we have commented where appropriate on specific screening procedures for school age children, the third edition focuses on the pre-school-age group. A detailed review of the health care needs of school-aged children will be found in the 1995 Polnay Report (see note 3, p. 107).

New terminology

General practitioners and health visitors have shown a considerable and increasing commitment to provision of a good CHS service. Nevertheless, the process of seeking for defects and disorders (secondary prevention) continues to receive a higher priority than primary prevention. This may reflect the differing emphasis given previously to these topics in the first two editions, where we devoted considerable space to the issue of screening and surveillance. Although we recognized that primary prevention and health promotion could be integrated into the programme of CHS, we did not address the topic in detail.

In order to emphasize that preventive health care for children involves more than the detection of defects, implied in the concept of surveillance, we propose that the 1996 programme should be called 'Child Health Promotion' (CHP). The term 'child health surveillance' (CHS) will be retained but will refer specifically to activities designed to achieve early detection ('secondary prevention').

How will the changes affect the Primary Health Care Team and the General Practitioner?

Although we hope that the 1996 programme will increase the emphasis on primary prevention, its delivery remains within the remit of the Primary Health Care Team. We have recommended some modifications to the content of child health surveillance, but the overall design of the programme is essentially the same as in our previous reports. We suggest a move towards increased flexibility, giving more scope for professional judgement as to what type and level of service is provided for each child and family.

Workload and resource implications

We did not anticipate, and do not envisage, that our proposals would increase the total time or resources committed to preventive child health. We recognize that the increased emphasis on primary prevention and health promotion might be perceived as an increase in workload. This is not the intention. Rather, we have tried to identify and separate out the various strands of current activity in preventive child health so that we could describe them in detail, just as we did for the various screening procedures in the first two editions of *Health for all children*. This task is an essential prelude to further audit, evaluation, and research.

CHP tasks, services and goals

Although these are not new, the level of commitment to these tasks has varied widely and there has in many districts been little attempt to specify aims or to measure improvements or outcomes. Examples of CHP include promotion of breast-feeding, by individual and peer support and by better maternity unit policies; identification and management of postnatal depression; measures to reduce child neglect and abuse, and unintentional injury; better immunization and immunization advice (particularly for BCG and hepatitis B uptake which audit has shown to be unsatisfactory in many districts); developmental and nutritional guidance, including dental care; special services for families with disabled children, ethnic minorities, etc. We suggest ways in which these activities might be monitored, and emphasize the implications for training.

Needs assessment and targeting

The identification of health care needs is central to CHP. It cannot be achieved by checklists or rigid guidelines; needs assessment requires the development of a relationship between parents and health care staff, and mature professional judgement. All families should have access to the full range of skills within the primary health care team but they vary widely in the level of professional support they need to achieve the goals of CHP. Only a minority need intensive support and help, for example to facilitate their child's development or reduce the risk of child abuse. As these goals are attainable only by intensive, high quality programmes, resources should where possible be 'targeted' to families with clearly identified needs. The identification of such families is made easier by local data on housing, poverty and deprivation, social needs, access to services, etc.

A health services partnership

Primary health care teams* are pivotal in the delivery of the 1996 programme. In order to achieve more precise definition of need and better targeting of resources, with positive discrimination in favour of preventive health care and health promotion, they will need to draw on the expertise and differing perspectives of paediatricians and specialists in public health medicine, nursing and health promotion.

Partnership with other agencies

Support and advice for parents on child development, behaviour and nutrition is an important part of CHP. These tasks are not the province of health professionals alone but should be planned and shared with colleagues in departments of social services and education, and the skills and enthusiasm of the voluntary sector should be harnessed.

Improvements in CHS

For each screening programme (hips, hearing, vision, heart, testes, growth monitoring) a **clear pathway of referral must be agreed and an**

* The term 'Primary Health Care Team' is defined on p. 16.

audit undertaken of the system as a whole. The experience of identification as a 'screen positive' must be followed by a seamless pathway to secondary and, if necessary, tertiary specialists.

Physical examination

Some forms of congenital heart disease (p. 96) will not be diagnosable in the first few days of life, and vigilance on the part of parents and professionals is essential. Auscultation of the heart after 6–8 weeks is part of routine clinical care but should not be regarded as a screening procedure.

Despite doubts about screening for congenital dislocation of the hip (p. 92), this should continue at present. We suggest that there should be one examination as soon as possible after birth, and a further examination at the review at 6–8 weeks is suggested. Ultrasound may be used for secondary screening at 2 weeks (preferably in the context of a clinical trial), but routine primary ultrasound screening (i.e. of all births) is not justified except for research. The hips should be checked again preferably at 6–9 months, but a check with the third immunization is an alternative possibility which deserves evaluation. The gait should be observed when the child starts to walk. Checks after the 6–8 week review do not currently meet the criteria for a screening test, and should be regarded as case finding.

If **testes** (p. 102) are not descended at the 6–8 week examination, the child should be referred to a surgeon with paediatric experience; ideally, he should be seen by the surgeon at around 6–9 months. Further screening checks are not justified.

Regular CHS reviews

There are various options for the neonatal examination (p. 90) including the possibility that midwives, with appropriate training, could undertake the task. The review recommended at **6–9 months** does not include any procedure which can be regarded as a formal screening procedure, apart from the hearing test (see below). Reviews at 1–2 years and at 3–3 years do not contain any formal screening procedures. There can and should be more flexibility in the level of professional input at these checks.

Growth monitoring

This term is better than growth screening (p. 109) because many growth problems are only detectable by measurements over a period of time. Length should be measured, *if indicated*, at 6–8 weeks. Height should be checked at around the ages of 1½–2, 3½, and 5 years (p. 109). A further measurement at about age 7 is proposed, but with certain caveats. We stress the need to assess the benefits of this programme and discuss the difficult problem of referral criteria (p. 124). The nine-centile charts should be used for all growth monitoring.

The clinical assessment of non-organic failure to thrive is difficult, and staff training is mandatory in order to ensure that problems are accurately identified and that the parents of normal small children are not worried unnecessarily (p. 112).

Hearing screening

The role of neonatal screening and of the distraction test at 6–8 months is still uncertain. We set out the options for screening programmes in the first year of life. Neonatal screening may turn out to be the best option but, for districts not yet committed to this approach, selective or high-risk screening is probably a better investment at present than universal screening (p. 151). The distraction test at 6–8 months only produces good results if training and monitoring are of a very high standard. Its place in districts with neonatal screening is still under debate (p. 153).

After the first year of life, we do not recommend any further universal 'intermediate' screening until school entry, but any child with developmental or behavioural problems should be considered for hearing assessment. Most important, *no* programme of screening is worthwhile unless it is supported by a well-run modern audiology clinic. Districts should review the overall quality of their audiology service for children *before* changing their screening programme.

Vision screening

Formal tests for squint and visual acuity are not recommended prior to school entry unless carried out by an orthoptist or other appropriately trained person (p. 168). We suggest that a community orthoptic service is likely to be cost-effective and should be provided, but it should be regarded as an outreach from the ophthalmology clinic rather than a true screening programme (p. 171).

Laboratory and radiological procedures

We recommend that responsibility for biochemical screening (phenylketonuria, hypothyroidism, etc.) should be clearly identified (p. 131). A policy should be established for screening for hypothyroidism in children with Down's syndrome (p. 132). There should be a formal multidisciplinary review of services for people with haemoglobinopathies; screening should be considered but in the context of an overall service review.

Iron deficiency

Iron deficiency (p. 140) is an important health problem in young children. It is more prevalent in some inner city areas and ethnic minorities, but can occur in all sectors of society. Screening programmes are feasible and are acceptable to the population at risk, but may not be the ideal solution. Enhanced efforts at primary prevention will probably turn out to be a more cost-effective approach.

Developmental reviews

As in previous editions, we recognize that this is still a contentious area. We have not found any reason to reverse our previous doubts about the value of routine developmental testing for all children. Instead, we suggest priorities for the detection of children with disabilities, environmental disadvantage affecting development, and severely impaired language and communication skills (p. 191). The identification of isolated delay in speech development ('expressive language') at the 2-year-old review is *not* regarded as a priority (p. 204). We provide a summary of knowledge about intervention for children with speech and language delay.

Child mental health

The primary care team has a potentially important role in preventing, identifying and managing straightforward behavioural difficulties (p. 199). Further training and better specialist support will be needed.

Information systems

Information systems need to be improved (p. 212). Each district needs a single database with demographic details and birth data for every child, the NHS number, and the post code. The system should eventually be linked to other health care provider information databases. We suggest that data items should only be collected on computer (either centrally or in primary care teams) if they meet strict criteria.

There is an increasing problem with litigation for conditions 'missed' by screening tests and for other potentially avoidable failures in preventive child health care. We list the areas which we regard as particular hazards.

Each district or health authority should appoint a steering group to oversee and the chairperson should be called the CHP Coordinator. The CHP policy statement should specify not only the procedures to be followed, but also referral pathways, quality of service to be provided for screen-positive individuals, data to be collected (including data relevant to health promotion), measures of improvement, and training requirements for staff (p. 217).

Personal child health records

Guidelines on the use of personal child health records are updated (p. 219). We stress the importance of clarifying the question of confidentiality and use of data when issuing these records.

1

Health for all children?

In this chapter, we shall:
- Outline the shift in emphasis from child health surveillance to child health promotion
- Define the terms used:
  Health promotion.
  Public policy issues
  Community development
  Health education
  Intervention
  Prevention (primary, secondary, and tertiary)
- Stress the need for an evidence-based service

The first edition of *Health for all children* set out a programme of routine reviews for all preschool children and subsequently, in a second edition, suggested how this might be delivered. This, the third edition, is a response to evolving professional perceptions of preventive health care, coupled with rapid changes in the political context in which that care is provided.

The theme of the third edition of *Health for all children* is child health promotion. Its message is that preventive health services for children extend beyond the narrow remit of child health surveillance, with its focus on the detection of abnormalities, to encompass positive efforts to prevent illness and promote good health. The term 'child health surveillance' will be redefined as 'activities related to secondary prevention', i.e. the detection of defects. Although important, it is not more important than the primary prevention of ill health. Thus, we shall regard child health surveillance as just one component of a Child Health Promotion programme.

The promotion of child health requires a shift in the relationship between parents, children, and health professionals to one of partnership rather than supervision, in which parents are empowered to make use of services and expertise according to their needs. Many professionals working with children have already embraced such working practices. This report reflects these changes, summarizes the strengths and weaknesses of the research evidence which underpins them, and suggests how further progress can be made.

Although some alterations have been proposed to the schedule of reviews and screening tests included in child health surveillance, these are less significant than the changes in the philosophy and the priorities set out in this report. The results of screening tests and checks are easier to record and measure than the activities and outcomes of health promotion, but this does not mean that they are more important. An increased emphasis on the promotion of health and on coordinated service provision will have implications for contracting and commissioning, service delivery, the structure of records, and the type of information which should be collected in order to monitor the programme.

Definitions and concepts

Precise definitions of the terms used in preventive child health care are essential before any attempt can be made to establish the nature of the task or the effectiveness of the activities involved. Definition of the terms 'health', 'health promotion', and 'child health surveillance' has been the source of much debate.[1]

Health promotion is 'any planned and informed intervention which is designed to improve physical or mental health or prevent disease, disability and premature death'. To avoid confusing the issues in child health with the controversies about adult health promotion by general practitioners, we shall use the term 'child health promotion' (CHP).

Child Health Promotion

Since health in childhood is affected not only by biological factors, but also by the lifestyle and problems of the parents, including unemployment, low income, and poor housing, CHP can encompass interventions in the following spheres: curative medicine, other facets of health services, efforts to provide a healthy social, physical, and work environment, education, and public policies affecting benefits, finance, employment, etc. Many of the measures which might improve health were considered to be outside the remit of the NHS until the recent reforms.

Until recently, much CHP has been based on the **preventive model** which aims at persuading parents to take responsible decisions and make changes to their lifestyle to benefit their children, for example stopping smoking. Its weakness is that it locates health problems at the level of the individual and appears to blame the victims for their ill health, ignoring the social and economic factors which often prevent people from making appropriate choices. For example, parents may be too poor to buy 'healthy' foods or recommended safety equipment.

In contrast, the **self-empowerment model** is concerned with 'empowering' people to achieve control over the factors which affect their lives.[2] This is achieved by the development of assertiveness and self-esteem at both individual and community level.

It is convenient to describe CHP as having the following components: public policy issues, advocacy, community development, health education, and clinical interventions, including disease prevention, at the individual level.

Public policy issues
Avoidable adverse health outcomes show a steep social class gradient[3] which is associated with undesirable living conditions, stress, and poverty (see box on p. 32). The level of investment in education also has implications for health in the widest sense, and for the identification and remediation of developmental problems in young children. Therefore the promotion of child health involves a range of legislative and policy initiatives, such as financial benefits, help for parents who experience conflicts between child care and the need to work, support for families of children with special needs, etc.

Health protection
Health protection refers to measures adopted to safeguard the health of the community as a whole: clean water, good sanitation, safe roads and playgrounds, housing policies that provide sufficient houses of adequate quality, etc. The term *Healthy Alliances* refers to collaboration between statutory agencies, voluntary bodies, and individuals in health protection, community development, and health education.

Housing problems
Poor housing is a major preoccupation for many parents. In some cases, health professionals are perceived as the route by which their housing needs can receive higher priority. Special pleas on behalf of individuals are useful only in exceptional circumstances. However,

health professionals can have a wider influence on local housing policy. For example, safety measures such as window locks can be introduced and standards for 'homeless family' accommodation can be established.

Advocacy

Advocacy is a long-established tool in public health. It means speaking out on behalf of a child, a family, or an issue such as the need for day nursery provision or legislation on tobacco advertising. It may be undertaken on behalf of individuals or communities, or nationally. It requires a good argument, persistence, and the avoidance of party political bias, together with an awareness of how the political system and the media operate.[4] It is more effective if a group of professionals speak with one voice.

Community development

Community development is the process by which local people define their own health needs and organize to make these needs known to service providers, or take action themselves in order to bring about change. This process may be facilitated by health professionals who can help to generate community interest in health, but it should not be dependent on them. Examples of community development projects include improvements in housing conditions, cleaning up local streets, and improving street lighting.

Health education

Health education is defined as 'any activity which promotes health through learning, i.e. some relatively permanent change in an individual's capabilities or dispositions'. It can be directed at individuals, groups or whole populations. It may incorporate the following.

- Basic biological knowledge of how the human body and mind work, how they can go wrong, and what can be done to maintain health. It may include information about child development, interactions within families, acquisition of child-rearing skills, etc.
- Consumer information on services and benefits.

• Personal strategies to cope with stress, loneliness, unemployment, poor housing, etc., and to develop assertiveness, individual strengths, and interests.

The first of these represents what most professionals have understood by health education, but a more modern view incorporates all three elements.

Clinical interventions with individual children and families

Intervention means activity initiated by a professional (or other individual outside the family) intended to deal with a problem affecting health or development. It should take account of the needs and views of the individual, and should aim to develop self-reliance rather than create dependence. It includes therapeutic services such as those provided by health care teams, hospital paediatric services, nursing, health visiting and midwifery, speech therapy, psychology, and other remedial professions, and educational and social work input as appropriate. Voluntary groups also contribute.

Community-based CHP projects

In addition to individual interventions with parents, group and community schemes contribute to the health of children. Examples include developing play schemes, drop-in centres, equipment stores, etc., changing attitudes in and access to local health services, and forming social and peer support groups for various activities. Effective projects may need to cross the traditional boundaries of primary health care teams or practice lists.

Disease prevention

Disease prevention has three components: primary, secondary, and tertiary.*

Primary prevention means the reduction of the number of new cases of a disease, disorder, or condition in a population, i.e. reduction of the **incidence**. It includes activities such as immunization, prevention of accidents and child abuse, advice and support for parents ('anticipatory guidance' in the US literature) dental prophylaxis, etc.

---

* The use of these terms does *not* imply that primary prevention is the task of primary health care teams or that secondary prevention is the province of specialists.

Secondary prevention is aimed at reducing the **prevalence** of disease and other departures from good health by shortening their duration or diminishing their impact through early detection and prompt and effective intervention. Inevitably, the distinction between primary and secondary prevention is hazy at times, particularly in the area of developmental and psychiatric disorders. *Screening* is just one of the means by which early identification can be achieved (p. 82).

Tertiary prevention is aimed at reducing impairments and disabilities, minimizing the suffering caused by existing departures from good health, and promoting the child's and parents' adjustment to conditions that cannot be ameliorated (Table 1.1).

Child health surveillance (CHS)

There is no uniformity in the definitions of CHS adopted by the many authorities who write on this subject. It has been used to include any or all of the following: the oversight of the physical, social, and emotional health and development of children, measurement and recording of physical growth, monitoring of developmental progress, offering and arranging intervention when necessary, prevention of disease by immunization and other means, and health education. The term has been used to denote not only the supervision of the health of the individual child, but also the process of monitoring the health of a whole community of children, by analogy with the public health function of monitoring the incidence of infectious diseases. We shall propose a definition that we believe will resolve these issues.

A *'seamless' service*: parents expect a high standard of clinical care throughout their contacts with the health services. The early identification of defects is of little value unless the parents subsequently experience a well-organized service from the first suspicion of a problem to definitive diagnosis and management. Screening and surveillance should no longer be commissioned in isolation from the clinical support required for effective care.

The term *'non-specific oversight'* means the vigilant supervision of all aspects of the health and well-being of children. We believe that this term is confusing and should be abandoned. The principle involved is incorporated in the wider concept of a health promotion programme.

The programme we shall recommend at the conclusion of our report should be regarded as a 'best buy' in the light of current evidence. We anticipate that it will continue to be refined and altered in the light of further research and experience.

Table 1.1   Terminology of impairment, disability, and handicap

A **disorder** is a medically definable condition or disease entity (*e.g. meningomyelocele*)

An **impairment** is any loss or abnormality of psychological, physiological, or anatomical structure or function (*e.g. paralysis of the legs*)

A **disability** is any restriction or lack (resulting from an impairment) of ability to perform an activity in the manner or within the range considered normal for a human being (*e.g. inability to walk*)

A **handicap** is the impact of the impairment or disability on the person's pursuit or achievement of the goals which are desired by him or expected of him by society (*e.g. unable to undertake any employment that requires mobility or access to public buildings*)

Mental impairment and learning disability There have been many changes over the years in the terminology used to describe children with low intellectual capacity, for example mental handicap, mental retardation, educational subnormality, etc. At present, the most widely used term in the UK is **learning disability**. We shall use the term **general (global) learning disability** to denote the presence of lower than normal intelligence (IQ) and **specific learning disability** for conditions such as reading impairment or 'dyslexia' where one particular function or skill is involved.

Changing terminology In recent years the international disability movements have emphasized the social, financial, and political aspects of disability, and various alternative uses of these terms have been proposed. For example, 'disability' rather than 'handicap' has been used to describe the total experience of being disabled, including the impact of the environment and the role of society. The term 'disadvantage' has also been proposed to encompass the negative effects of discrimination against disabled people. Nevertheless, the definitions given are still generally accepted by most health professionals in the UK, and we do not think that they should be abandoned until agreement can be reached on an alternative terminology.

The debate over terminology reflects a deeper dissatisfaction about attitudes to disability. The 'medical model' of disability, which locates the 'problem' within the individual, is caricatured as being obsessed with the pursuit of normality, the search for the perfect body and mind. It is a 'personal tragedy theory', a restricted view of disability as some terrible misfortune which occurs at random to certain individuals. In contrast, the 'social model of disability' locates the problem in society. Individual limitations are acknowledged but are seen as less important than society's failure to ensure that the needs of disabled people are taken into account in its organizations and facilities.

Terminology derived from *International Classification of Impairments, Disabilities and Handicaps*, WHO, Geneva, 1980.
Reproduced with permission from D.M.B. Hall and P. Hill (1995) *The child with a disability*, Blackwell, Oxford.

Public health

Reduction of health hazards and promotion of good health for all children involves not only 'traditional' one-to-one professional contacts but also a range of community-based measures. Some of these are aimed at the whole population of children; others are targeted to specific groups who are considered to be at increased risk or to have additional or complex needs. There are also families who are difficult to reach with routine services and need special provision, for example children of travelling families, the homeless, refugees, and Armed Forces personnel.

Identification of these groups is an essential public health task. Public health medicine aims to provide a collective view of health needs and health care of a population.[5] It can be defined as 'the science and art of preventing disease, prolonging life, and promoting health through the organized efforts of society' (see Table 1.2).

Responsibility for a population perspective is not exclusive to departments of public health medicine or community paediatricians but is shared with primary health care teams (PHCTs).* Members of the PHCT increasingly act as important agents for introducing and monitoring public health measures.

The need for an evidence-based child health service

It will probably never be possible to make recommendations which are wholly based on scientific considerations. There are some aspects of preventive child health work which will always be difficult to measure. The value of some services is supported by persuasive evidence, whereas for others the evidence is insufficient to make any firm judgement. When resources are limited, they should be devoted to activities where the maximum health gain seems likely to be achieved. At the same time, the concerns and preoccupations of parents must be considered; services perceived as valuable by the 'consumer' should not be too readily dismissed even if evidence of effectiveness is scanty. For

---

* The 'primary health care team' is generally taken to mean the general practitioner, health visitor, practice nurse, district nurse, practice manager, and ancillary staff, but the Working Party believes that, for the purposes of CHP, the term could usefully be broadened to include others who contribute to the primary care of children, for example community health doctors, community orthoptists, audiometricians, and so on. This report uses the term 'primary health care team' to encompass all such staff.

Table 1.2 Responsibilities of public health[5]

- Monitoring and describing the health of the population
- Identifying those groups most in need of health care of all kinds and most likely to benefit from health care
- Identifying the social, economic, and environmental factors that impinge on health
- Taking action to promote and improve health
- Assessing the impact of health care interventions on the health of the population

example, continuity of care and advice is rated highly by many service users.

The need for innovation and experiment

In many districts, there will be one or more services which are not specified in our list of recommendations. *Provided that* (a) the justification for these is clearly articulated and (b) useful data are being collected, we would regard such services as a valuable 'natural experiment'. Purchasers should not discontinue these but rather should consider them as a means of increasing the national pool of knowledge. Districts with innovative approaches to child health promotion and surveillance may in due course find that they have a valuable resource of clinical and technological expertise. Peer review may help to ensure that the maximum benefit is obtained from these programmes.

Recommendations

- We propose that the **overall programme of child care should be identified and planned as a 'Child Health Promotion (CHP) Programme'.** This term would be more in keeping with current thinking abut the nature of health, the central role of parents, and the importance of parent 'empowerment'.
- **Child Health Surveillance should be regarded as synonymous with secondary prevention and as one component of CHP.** This suggestion was made originally by Butler and should be adopted. We recognize that the term 'child health surveillance' is so well established in the literature, and in the 1990 General Practitioner Contract, that these

re-definitions may cause some difficulty, but they do reflect important philosophical changes.

- The routine reviews and immunizations which should be available to all children were called the '**core programme**' in the first two editions and we propose that this term should be retained. Some CHP messages are universally important and should be incorporated in the core programme.

- **The 'public health' responsibility for the health of all the children in a community should be shared between public health departments, paediatric services and primary health care teams.** Where appropriate, contracts should reflect the need to carry out community work with individuals or groups who receive their routine health care from other primary care teams.

- Commissioners and purchasers should require that **contracts for surveillance and screening programmes should incorporate appropriate secondary and, if necessary, tertiary care.** Monitoring and audit should consider the complete service and not focus solely on the detection process.

Notes and references

1. Terminology is discussed in Stone, D.H. (1990). Terminology in Community Child Health – an urgent need for consensus. *Archives of Disease in Childhood* **65**, 792–5. See also Tones, K., Tilford, S., and Robinson, Y. (1990). *Health education: effectiveness and efficiency*. Chapman & Hall, London; Dines, A. and Cribb, A. (1993). *Health promotion concepts and practice*. Blackwell, Oxford. For an excellent overview of evaluation methodology see Hawe, P., Degeling, D., and Hall, J. (1990). *Evaluating health promotion*. MacLennan & Petty, Sydney.
2. Gibson, C. (1991). A concept analysis of empowerment. *Journal of Advanced Nursing*, **16**, 354–61.
3. Black, D. (1980). *Inequalities in health*, HMSO, London.
4. Chapman, S. and Lupton, D. (1994). *The fight for the public health: principles and practice of media advocacy*. BMJ, London.
5. Committee of Enquiry into the Future Development of the Public Health Function (1988). *Public health in England*. HMSO, London.

2

Child health promotion

This chapter:
- considers the background of, and justification for, CHP
- describes the problems of demonstrating the efficacy of CHP
- discusses the role of health visitors and other professionals in taking responsibility for CHP
- examines the concept of 'needs assessment'
- reviews the tasks of CHP and evidence for the efficacy of individual CHP aims
- reviews the effectiveness of health-visiting programmes as a whole
- summarizes the lessons learned from the research review
- considers the implications of the research evidence for the provision of CHP services.
- makes recommendations for services and for further research

---

At first glance the aim of preventing illness and promoting good health does not seem to require any justification. Most parents want to make a success of bringing up their children, and many welcome help and guidance provided that it is given in a sensitive manner. Parents can feel inadequate and isolated, and are often subjected to poor advice from a variety of sources, yet they may feel reticent about asking for information and help. This chapter develops the point already made, that effective health promotion involves more than just giving information or offering help. It then reviews the effectiveness of CHP and emphasizes the importance of ensuring that it is delivered in a cost-effective way.

Although the health of children is first and foremost a parental responsibility, health professionals are expected to take an active interest in promoting children's health. Society has a vested interest in ensuring that the rights and needs of children are respected. This can be expressed in many ways, including legislation, improvement of the environment, appropriate health services, and financial benefits.

Nevertheless, health professionals must always consider whether they have a mandate to intrude on the life of any individual in order to promote his or her health. Health care staff (who are predominantly white and middle class) do not have a monopoly of wisdom in matters of child care, child rearing, or family life. The insights of developmental psychology, linguistics, and child psychiatry do not guarantee that we now know the 'right' or 'best' way to bring up children. Unsolicited advice may not always be welcome.[1]

In the UK, the historical context of health visiting, coupled with public and professional anxiety about child abuse and neglect, can result in the role of health promoter being confused with that of social worker, police officer, hygiene inspector, or NSPCC officer. Although health visitors are usually welcomed by parents, the professional expectation that they can be relied on to identify child abuse can place them in a difficult position.[2] (This is less of a problem in countries such as France, where the division of responsibility between health visitor and social worker is much sharper and there is more support for families with young children, so that their care is shared between parents and other adults.[3])

Whose responsibility?

Responsibility for CHP is shared between primary health care teams, midwives, paediatricians, and public health staff, in addition to specialists in CHP working in health promotion units. Many of the aims of CHP overlap with those of the education and social services. Other local authority departments, for example those responsible for housing, roads, and playgrounds, should also be involved. The media play an increasingly active role. Since so many individuals and disciplines are involved in the promotion of health, shared planning, consistent advice, and honesty about areas of uncertainty are vital.

Hospital staff share responsibility for CHP—it is not solely a community-based task. There are numerous opportunities for promoting health in hospital practice, including giving immunizations during hospital admissions, ensuring follow-up from the accident and emergency department after children's accidents (for example using liaison health visitors), and developing community paediatric nursing services to minimize the impact of childhood illnesses.

The emphasis on health visiting in the following discussion does not mean that this is the only discipline with an interest in or responsibility for health-promoting activities. Nevertheless, in the UK health visitors are closely identified with CHP, particularly with preschool children, and much of the relevant research involves assessment of health-visiting practice, both in the UK and overseas.[4] In the North American literature the term 'home visitation' is used; in some countries, the nurse is called an MCH (maternal and child health) nurse.

The tasks of health promotion

The tasks of CHP are summarized in Table 2.1.

Needs assessment

This term is used in various ways by the different disciplines involved in child health. It is important to distinguish between the public health function of assessing the health needs of populations and the responsibility of individual practitioners to assess the health and health care needs of their clients and case loads.

Determining health care needs
Identifying needs for health care and stimulating awareness of health care needs are two key elements of health-visiting practice. More

Table 2.1

- **Needs assessment:** determining the need for CHP is an essential prelude to the tasks described below.
- **Emotional support:** by listening, sharing experiences, providing counselling for depression and mood disorders, friendship, introductions to other people in similar circumstances, formation of groups.
- **Provision of education:** by information (written, spoken, media, video, etc.), demonstration, or role modelling.
- **Prevention and detection of disorders and health problems**
- **Practical help:** crisis assistance, introduction to services, help with transport, interpreting, advocacy, and specific health care measures which are difficult for some individuals to access (e.g. home immunization of a child where the parent is disabled or agoraphobic).
- **Community-based projects** such as equipment loan schemes.
- **Community development** as outlined on p. 12.

---

research is required on how, and how effectively, this is done. Although various attempts have been made to create checklists that might facilitate recognition of 'vulnerable' or 'high-risk' families, this approach does not seem to have any beneficial effect on health care, resource allocation, or outcome. There are probably several reasons for this.

First, there is no agreed definition of what is meant by 'vulnerable' or 'high risk'.[5] To some staff, these terms are more or less synonymous with being 'at risk' of abuse or neglect. To others, the concept has a much wider meaning and includes those children who would be regarded as 'children in need' under the 1989 Children Act and others who are perceived as needing extra help. 'Vulnerability' might be a permanent state for a few families, but for many others it is transient and changes with life circumstances and events. This may in part explain why scoring systems to identify parents of newborn infants who are at risk of abusing their child have limited predictive power.

Second, health professionals develop an intuitive sense about the health and the needs of their patients or clients,[6] and this is probably more sensitive than any checklist. This intuition is based on knowledge and experience, familiarity with a family's previous history, and an understanding of the local neighbourhood. Stress factors may be internal (depression, poor health, disabled child) or external (housing problems, financial difficulties). Checklists may overemphasize vulnerability factors and ignore protective resources, such as a supportive partner or a close relationship with a friend or relative, yet the latter are at least as important in determining needs.[7] The weight which should be attached to each adverse and protective factor would have to be fixed in a formal checklist approach, but can be assessed individually by an experienced professional.

Third, although some needs may be identified by the parent or obvious to the professional, some problems are only identified by leading questions and may be acknowledged by the parent only after a relationship with the professional has been established. Sensitivity is essential in raising personal matters—this cannot easily be done in one visit or by using a formal checklist.

What determines the effectiveness of individual health care needs assessment?
This is dependent on a number of factors.

1. It is essential that staff have the time and the skills to listen to what parents are saying and try to develop a genuine sense of partnership, rather than imposing their own agenda or that of their managing authority.

2. All professionals need to be aware of, and resist, the tendency to assess and act on the perceived 'social worth' of patients and clients. 'Worth' in this sense does not refer to their social status; it is a more complicated concept involving estimates of how deserving the client is of help, whether their needs are a legitimate call on the professional's time, and whether the client is responsive to the offers made by the professional.[8]

3. Health professionals are often wary of discussing needs for which no service exists, particularly if, as is often the case, they have no direct means of influencing the planning of services. In this situation, it is important that unmet needs *are* acknowledged, documented, and brought to the attention of purchasers, public health physicians, and other relevant authorities. This advocacy role may not be perceived as important or effective by the family concerned but its long-term benefits should be stressed (see Chapter 1, p. 12).

4. Alternatively, there is a risk that clients may be matched to the service which comes closest to meeting their needs, even if it is not the ideal. Health professionals may be tempted to construe problems in terms of health care needs that *can* be met by the health service, when sometimes other solutions might be more appropriate. This can result in disappointment and time-wasting for the individual, and reduces the efficiency of the service in question.

5. Cultural, religious, ethnic, and language barriers may prevent accurate needs assessment in precisely those families who are likely to benefit most from a variety of different services.[9]

6. Children's own perceptions of need are often ignored or are not taken seriously.[10] It is important that professionals learn to listen to children's concerns, particularly in situations that may cause additional stress (e.g. children who are acting as carers).

The importance of support and counselling

Social support and the development of good relationships with individual parents and families is not only worthwhile for its own sake but is also an essential prelude to effective health promotion.

Health professionals sometimes regard 'support' as a 'soft' concept—
an activity not worth measuring or purchasing. Nevertheless there is a
substantial body of research on the subject. Support can be defined as
'information leading the subject to believe that he or she is cared for,
loved, esteemed, and a member of a network of mutual obligations'.

The ability of individuals to cope with stress varies considerably. In
addition to intrinsic factors, such as mental resilience, temperament,
and physical health and endurance, external factors play a part in
determining which parent will succumb to stress and which will sur-
vive. These include, for example, the influence of family, friends, and
neighbours, the availability of other interested adults to befriend the
children, and the quality of local schooling.

Social support is one way of reducing the stress of disadvantage,
social isolation, and hopelessness which characterizes many deprived
populations and affects every aspect of life, including motivation for
care of self and family and the ability to be a 'good enough' parent.
Support improves pregnancy outcomes,[11] reduces depression in vulnerable women,[12] enables mothers to provide more stimulation for their
children, and reduces the risk of child abuse and neglect.

Individuals turn first for support to family and friends, and subsequently to a range of people encountered during everyday life.
Together, these form a social support network—a 'set of intercon-
nected relationships among a group of people who provide enduring
patterns of nurturance and reinforcement for efforts to cope with
everyday life'. Some networks are informal, some are contrived
extended families, and some are created in response to a common life
situation or crisis.[13]

Formal professional help may be sought, but most individuals are
reluctant to disclose their problems and concerns to a stranger unless
an empathic trusting relationship exists or can be created. It takes time
to develop such relationships. The role of the professional is to identify
need, facilitate the development of support networks, and provide support personally for individuals who for various reasons, such as loneliness or depression, are unable to build other relationships.

Counselling is a means to an end. It can be defined* as 'an interaction in which one person offers another time, attention and respect
with the intention of helping that person to explore, discover and clarify
ways of living more successfully and to his/her greater wellbeing'.
Good listening, communicating, and note-taking skills are central to

* British Association for Counselling.

any CHP activity with individuals. These skills can be taught and improvements can be measured.[14] Effective counselling is inhibited by the pressure to cover a wide range of health care issues in a short time, particularly when the concerns of the individual do not coincide with the agenda of the professional, manager, or commissioner/ purchaser.

Meeting the needs of various ethnic groups

Service provision for other ethnic groups is important if the needs of all children are to be met. Provision of special programmes for conditions such as sickle cell disease is a necessary but not sufficient response to the needs of ethnic groups. Other requirements may include linkworker schemes, dieticians with special knowledge of weaning and feeding practices, translations of written information, local radio health programmes, etc. Information and advice must be culturally sensitive and relevant. Staff need to understand the attitudes, customs, and communication styles of the groups with whom they work, and to recognize the dangers of stereotyping members of ethnic groups.

The problem of low literacy

Estimates of illiteracy and of problems with reading and writing vary, but perhaps 10 per cent of the population may have such difficulties. The implications of this are often forgotten. Many people will be unable to benefit from written material even at a simple level, yet much health promotion literature requires a sophisticated level of reading skill and excellent reading comprehension. Readability scores provide an objective method of assessment. The production of more accessible materials and a review of existing literature, posters, etc. should be a priority. Collaborations with Adult Education Units may be one way to proceed. Useful guidance has been published by the Health Education Board for Scotland.

Written information

The use of leaflets and information sheets must not be equated with health promotion. Careful design and explanation of the contents are essential. This applies as much to the personal child health record as to any other written material.

Practical help

Examples were given in Table 2.1. There are many situations where such help is the only way to ensure that children receive the medical or social care they need.

The role of non-qualified staff ('paraprofessionals')

Professionals are not essential in every situation.[15] The needs of some families can be met as effectively, or in some cases more effectively, by non-qualified or lay staff. This has obvious advantages; individuals can be selected from their own community, and therefore are familiar with its lifestyle and its problems, and they bring an income into their family and into their community.

Not surprisingly, this option has attracted much interest for both financial and philosophical reasons. Nevertheless, it is not necessarily a simple or cheap option. To be successful, paraprofessional staff need training and support; their case-loads are usually smaller than those of professionals, but their ability to cope with stressful problems may be reduced, particularly if they themselves are subject to similar life stresses. Some families may be reluctant to disclose problems to lay workers (though others may be equally reluctant with professionals). Lay workers and the members of voluntary organizations such as Homestart or Newpin (p. 72) provide a valuable service and should be encouraged and supported. They are neither a threat to nor a substitute for professionals.

Those parents who would have the most to gain from social support networks and lay worker schemes are often the least accessible and amenable to receiving help unless someone (usually a professional) leads them into participation. Social networks require that everyone has something of value to give in return for what he or she receives. 'People solve personal problems, accomplish tasks, develop social competence and address issues through an exchange of resources with members of their community. This exchange of resources . . . can be tangible goods like information or money, or intangible like emotional nurturance . . . .' People who are heavily in debt to their network may cut themselves off or be cut off from future transactions. 'A professional may need to restart the process for a bankrupt member of the network[13].'

What is the relationship between Child Health Surveillance and Child Health Promotion?

For many years, the early identification of disorders and defects was seen as a central task of community child health services and occupied a substantial proportion of health professionals' time. It received a correspondingly prominent position in the first and second editions of *Health for all children*. The task is indeed important, but detection of defects constitutes secondary prevention ('surveillance' in the terminology proposed on p. 17) and should not take precedence over primary prevention.

The core programme of reviews and checks at specified ages, set out in previous editions of *Health for all children*, is thought to be valuable, not only because previously unsuspected problems may be found, but for several other reasons.

• It provides a framework which encourages formation of a constructive relationship between professional and family, allowing the promotion of health independent of the stress caused by acute medical problems.

• It provides opportunities for health education and guidance which can be linked to developmental stages (for example accident prevention).

• It provides a flexible framework of reviews and advice which can be delivered in various ways and with varying levels of professional input according to the needs of the family.

• It reduces the chances of families with unrecognized needs being 'missed' by the network of services.

• It provides a convenient vehicle for securing high uptake of immunizations.

The value of early detection of disorders and defects is discussed in more detail in Chapter 5.

Ethical considerations

Like any other health care intervention, CHP has the potential to do harm as well as good. The information offered may turn out to be inaccurate or incorrect. Health information may cause anxiety or guilt to individuals who for various reasons cannot act on the advice given.

Whereas the individual who has a health problem can decide what to disclose to his or her chosen medical adviser, and whether to accept the treatment offered, it may be difficult to avoid CHP information. There is, therefore, an ethical imperative to ensure that CHP activities are subjected to as robust an evaluation as any other health care intervention.

Problems in the evaluation of CHP

The aims of CHP are admirable but, as with other aspects of child health care, it is important to marshall evidence of effectiveness and to establish how this can be monitored and, where possible, increased. The evidence that CHP can be effective is robust in some fields (e.g. prevention of infectious diseases), suggestive in others (e.g. accident prevention), and only preliminary in a few (e.g. prevention of child mental health problems).[16]

In reviewing the functions, effectiveness, and future role of preventive services for children, we were confronted by a number of difficulties which are less prominent in other aspects of health care research.

- Many of the tasks and activities involve several different disciplines within the NHS (for example community doctors, health visitors, general practitioners, and speech therapists). Each of these has different perspectives on assessment and management. Many activities also involve collaboration with other agencies such as the social services, education, and housing departments, the police, the NSPCC, etc. Therefore the effectiveness of health professionals is inextricably linked with that of other agencies.

- In many cases the important outcome measures can only be determined many years into the future. For example, detection and treatment of a conductive hearing defect in infancy might result in educational benefit when the child is 5 or 10 years old.

- The services provided are not glamorous or high profile, and many are concerned with prevention rather than curative medicine. This means that public demand is limited, research funding is not easy to obtain, and the level of service required must be defined by professional assessment of need. Attitudes are now changing, in line with new professional and governmental priorities but it will take many years to generate the necessary research base.

- Collection of the information required to assess and monitor preventive child health services is difficult because of the many sites where the services are delivered (homes, schools, clinics, nurseries, etc). Problems with computer databases in child health continue to limit the comparison of data between districts.

- Most health promotion involves three levels of input: legislation, local government initiatives, or community pressure to bring about changes in the environment or in products; advertising (written information, television campaigns, videos, etc.), which provides information and influences behaviour; education at the level of the individual or community-based group. The effects are synergistic, and attempts to measure them separately are fraught with difficulty. The introduction of seat-belt legislation, the change in society's attitude to drunken driving, and the decline in smoking rates provide excellent examples of successful but multifaceted campaigns.[17]

- Some of the adverse outcomes which health promotion activities may seek to prevent are rare, so that very large samples are needed to measure effectiveness directly. For example, sudden infant death is rare in an individual district. It may be necessary to use proxy measures; for example, the number of parents who place their babies to sleep in the supine position can be assessed at local level but the impact on the rate of sudden infant death can only be measured in much larger populations.

- Health professionals will vary in their skill in health promotion and in their impact on individual parents. Thus caution is necessary when generalizing from a research study to other situations. It is essential to maintain enthusiasm and to provide regular feedback and updates, otherwise even the most effective measures may lose their impact.

- Some alterations in health-related behaviour only occur gradually, and may depend on cultural changes or on shifts in the parents' own expectations of health and of the health-care system. The time span may be too long for changes to be identified within the scope of a research programme.

- 'Quick fix' solutions may look tempting, yet may not necessarily offer the best long-term answer to a problem. For an example, see the discussion on iron deficiency anaemia (p. 140).

- Much research has ignored the influence of fathers.[18] Their views are often neglected, and they are often marginalized in health promotion with young families. Similarly, the views of children themselves are seldom sought—even though it is their health which is being promoted! Addressing these issues is difficult even if one subscribes to the principle.

Evidence of effectiveness—lessons from the literature review

Evidence of effectiveness was considered under the following headings:

- Evaluation of specific programmes and activities; for example, prevention of accidents caused by falling from the windows of tall buildings (p. 48).
- Evaluation of programmes with a set of closely related aims, for example measuring the effect of an intensive campaign to reduce a range of childhood accidents (p. 47).
- Evaluation of programmes with more wide-ranging aims, for example the studies carried out by Olds[19] (p. 71).

The findings are cited in the relevant sections of this book. Although the evidence is incomplete, and involves many different cultures and populations, a number of themes have emerged which we believe are sufficiently robust to inform future planning of health promotion services for children and young families. One clear message is that services which are highly rated by parents have certain characteristics in common (see Table 2.2).

Secondly, even when the criteria in Table 2.2 are fulfilled, as in demonstration projects and research studies, the benefits, though statistically significant and valuable in economic terms, are modest in magnitude. It is reasonable to suppose that the benefits will be even smaller for programmes of lesser quality and intensity. We shall argue from this that doing some things well and in depth for some individuals is likely to be more cost effective than providing a token service to a large number of people.

Thirdly, health education which overloads the parent with too many messages is ineffective. It may be necessary to *create* an interest in CHP topics which are perceived by the parent as irrelevant to their life situa-

Table 2.2 Characteristics of successful programmes and projects

- Services are broad spectrum and comprehensive, crossing traditional professional boundaries, and are coherent and easy to use
- Both the structure and the individual staff are flexible in their ability to respond to unexpected demands
- The staff have both the time and the skill to establish a relationship of respect and trust with families
- The child is seen as a member of the family, and the family as part of a community
- Projects have enthusiastic committed leadership, clearly specified measurable aims and focus on families with high levels of need (typically poor, unsupported, and young, or having children with special problems)
- There is sustained high quality of input and, importantly, sufficient *continuity* of input to develop a relationship with the individual client (in many cases this implies commencing a professional relationship during pregnancy rather than after the child is born).

Derived from Larner, M. *et al.* (1992). *Fair start for children. Lessons learned from seven demonstration projects.* Yale University Press.[15]

tion. A 'curriculum' or agenda of parent education may be helpful, but is unlikely to bring about changes in lifestyle and parent practices unless a relationship is developed over a period of time:

. . . parent educators do not add information into a void. Parents sort, fit and modify new information according to their assumptions, values and levels of reasoning about parent-child relationships.[20]

Fourthly, an understanding of poverty and deprivation is central to planning CHP.[21] This is a complex issue and the temptation to stereotype must be avoided. Families regarded as having high levels of need because of poverty, disability, illness, membership of minority groups, etc, are not homogeneous. They are very diverse, differing in lifestyle, support networks, and beliefs. Some have had so many life disappointments that they are very difficult to engage in any useful professional contact (for example, those who have had no employment for two or even three generations). Others, though poor and under privileged, hope that their children may have a better life and have the personal capacity to work for this. This applies, for example, to many first-generation immigrants and to many refugees.[22]

In industrialized countries, the effect of relative poverty is probably more important than absolute income (see box). The pressures of consumerism and the sense of personal hardship and deprivation engendered by advertising may play some part in this.

... The sense of relative deprivation, of being at a disadvantage in relation to those better off, probably extends far beyond the conventional boundaries of poverty. A shift in emphasis from absolute to relative standards indicates a fall in the importance of the direct physical effects of material circumstances relative to psycho-social influences. The social consequences of people's differing circumstances in terms of stress, self-esteem and social relations may now be one of the most important influences on health.

R. Wilkinson, Income distribution and life expectancy,
British Medical Journal, **304**, 165 (1992)

By necessities, I understand not only the commodities which are indispensably necessary for the support of life, but whatever the custom of the country renders it indecent for creditable people, even of the lowest order, to be without.

Adam Smith, *The wealth of nations* (1776)

The health care system does not easily adapt to the needs of such families. Poor families may not seek help when it is needed. They may be less able to cope with internal and external pressures, and are often preoccupied with problems of money, housing, or work, so that health checks for apparently healthy children may have low priority. Lack of transport and telephones results in missed appointments, which irritates professionals and is often misinterpreted as indifference or neglect. Parents and children are difficult to visit at home because they are out at work or seeking work, they move frequently, and the child may be with a childminder or the extended family for a large part of the day. In some cultures teenage parents may share responsibility for childcare with their parents.

The families at greatest risk are 'outside the system'; this includes alcohol and drug abusers, victims of domestic violence, many homeless families, refugees, and some with unorthodox lifestyles. They do not seek help; they cannot handle the bureaucracy and perceived middle-class orientation of the health care system, and they find that public services are largely irrelevant to their lives. Understandably, such families are often suspicious of professionals and may see them as inspectors, or as representatives of the police or social services.

Nevertheless, only a small minority of parents neglect or abuse their children. Most are concerned about their child's health and progress, and the majority welcome advice and guidance. Concerns about 'bad' behaviour, learning difficulties, and social skills are common. For instance, parents worry about whether their child will make satisfactory progress when he or she starts school. If the child is slower than average, anxiety about the possible need for a 'special school' may be an important issue. When offered the opportunity, most parents, even in the poorest areas, appreciate guidance as to how they can help their child with reading and other schoolwork. Professionals are often reluctant to accept this interest and harness it.

Amidst concerns about deprivation, it is easy to overlook the concerns of middle-class parents. Such parents are perhaps more able to find solutions to their problems with a minimum of professional help, for example by establishing and maintaining contacts with peer groups. Nevertheless, divorce, financial problems, and ill health can be devastating for them, too. They may need help with concerns about issues such as promoting child mental health and managing behaviour or learning and language problems. Even parents who are highly educated are sometimes surprisingly uninformed about child development and the limits of normality.

Implications for CHP—targeting and its problems

We have argued that resources will be used more effectively if the aims are specified and target populations are clearly identified. The aims of CHP should be the same for all parents, but they may be achieved in various ways. Some parents will need considerable personal help either at specific times or for a continuous period; others need only appropriate information and ready access to professional advice when they have concerns.

Decisions about targeting must be made at three different levels:

- in the geographic sense—some parts of a health district will have much higher levels of need than others;
- Within the case-loads or practices of individual practitioners or PHCTs.

• in working with individual families or small groups, it may be necessary to focus on particular themes and problems and to defer others
which have a lower priority, as discussed previously.

Geographic and PHCT targeting

Information about the relative needs of different areas of a district is
required. Assessing these needs is a complex and potentially time-
consuming undertaking. It is only worthwhile if there is a commitment
to action. For example, many districts have a stated policy of positive
action in favour of the poorest areas in the use of community health
care resources.

However, inability to initiate staff redistribution, difficulties with
recruitment and morale in the most needy areas, and distortions introduced by changing patterns of funding often result in no net change or
even an increase in resource allocation to more prosperous areas.

The exercise known as community profiling can facilitate decision
making about targeting, promote teamwork, and provide an information base on the health of children for practitioners and purchasers.[23] It
involves identification of factors that affect their health, and reviewing
access to and availability of statutory and voluntary services. The views
of local residents should be ascertained.

At community level, local and national data should be used together
with information on demographic and social characteristics, health status,
statutory and voluntary services, transport, and the physical environment. This can be analysed according to electoral ward or enumeration
district, health localities, or primary care team boundaries. Further
work is required to develop systems that can generate and utilize this
data more easily.[24]

Individual families

Assessment of the needs of a family can rarely be undertaken in a single
short visit or consultation, particularly when the parents are dealing
with their first child.[25] Families under stress may have difficulty in
deciding what their priorities are, and until they have built up a relationship with the professional it will be difficult to negotiate any firm
arrangements. Some factors (Table 2.3) in the parent(s) or child are
likely to increase the need as perceived by professionals (though not

Table 2.3 Examples of situations where increased support from health professionals may be indicated

- First pregnancies and first-time parents
- Breastfeeding mothers
- Mothers recovering from difficult delivery (e.g. Caesarean section), or suffering post-natal depression or mood disorders, particularly if the partner is unhelpful or absent, or the mother is lacking in other social support networks
- Unsupported young poor parent, particularly in substandard housing; any family in temporary accommodation.
- Domestic violence, drug or alcohol misuse
- Concern about possible child neglect or abuse; past or present concerns identified by the child protection system.
- Parent(s) with learning disability, poor skills in managing their affairs, lacking in confidence or with low self-esteem.
- Disabled parent—child has to be 'carer'.
- Child who is premature, low birth-weight, disabled, or chronically sick
- History of previous 'cot death' or other infant death
- Infant with 'difficult' temperament, irregular sleep patterns, difficult feeding, etc.
- Families with particular difficulties or combinations of problems in accessing services, e.g. mother tongue not English, combined with socio-economic disadvantage.
- Children Looked After by foster parents.

necessarily by parents). However, the needs of other families must not be neglected just because they are not included in a list of 'high-risk' factors or the family did not score sufficiently highly on a risk-scoring system to merit professional intervention.

Protocols which specify that certain parents must receive a certain level of input are naive since they fail to take account of (a) the parents' own wishes and their right to be involved in planning the health care support that they want, and (b) the other supporting resources available within and outside the family. There must be sufficient flexibility for health professionals to negotiate the optimal care programme and to increase or reduce their involvement according to need.

It is important to remember the potential hazards of targeted CHP services. By focusing too closely on specific groups of parents, particularly if defined in terms of poverty or dependency needs, there is a risk that the provision of CHP services will become in itself a stigmatizing action. It would be most unfortunate if regular visits by a health professional were to be seen as evidence of being a bad parent.

These hazards can largely be avoided if (a) a minimum level of contact is offered for all families, as recommended in the core programme set out on p. 223, (b) the CHP programme and the roles of the health visitor and other professionals are presented in a positive light, and (c) the individual needs of each family are reviewed and negotiated openly with the parents. The personal child health record offers a useful way of ensuring that these requirements are being fulfilled.

Flexibility—using the telephone
In order to make optimum use of time, PHCT staff must be free to increase the intensity of support to families in need; conversely, they may be able to reduce the input to families who have no particular needs or problems. In the latter case, telephone calls are used in some districts to maintain contact with the family. Telephone interpreter services are an efficient way of ensuring that health care staff can communicate effectively with non-English speakers, removing the need for the interpreter to visit the family home. This approach has been used very effectively in Australia.

Recommendations—the key aims

1. **The Core Programme of Child Health Surveillance** consists of a series of routine reviews designed to achieve early identification and referral of children with developmental disorders and health problems together with information about the aims of the CHP programme. **This should be available to every parent.**

2. As a prelude to CHP, the **health care needs of each family with a new infant should be determined.** The level of professional input to the CHP programme need not and should not be the same for every family. It should be based on evaluation of the differing needs of localities and individuals. Families whose situation changes should be offered a review of their needs.

3. **The impact on the child of parental depression, disability, mood disorder, or social isolation should be minimized by the provision of appropriate advice and support.** Training programmes and packages are available to help health visitors and other professionals deal with these problems more effectively.

4. **Resource allocation** should take the following into account:
   - The needs of special groups (p. 57).
   - The need for intensive high-quality specialized services for carefully selected individuals. These may need additional skills and resources, and often involve other agencies.
   - The investment of time required to develop locally based community CHP projects and, where appropriate, to undertake community profiling.
5. It is essential to establish and maintain an **effective infrastructure**: for example, easy access to clinics and other centres, ready availability of education materials, flexibility in deciding which families need home visits, links with other educational services and opportunities (e.g. local radio), development of Healthy Alliances (p. 11), and an epidemiological information system.
6. **Monitoring and management** systems should measure only those parameters which are useful. Numbers of contacts are of minimal value; the aim should be to maximize the time spent in individual and group work with parents and children.

Research and development

- The literature on CHP overlaps with that of many other disciplines. Multidisciplinary literature reviews would be valuable to cross existing professional boundaries.
- Continuing research on the content, effectiveness, and health economics of methods of delivery CHP is essential. This is particularly important with regard to ethnic groups, people with literacy problems, and communities with special needs and problems.
- The immediate challenge is to develop a formal yet flexible framework for targeting resources, and then to find ways whereby the aims, activities, and results of health promotion can be monitored by both individual health professionals and departments of public health without increasing the time spent in record keeping (see p. 215). Better process and outcome measures, and improved information systems are needed.
- More work is required on involving fathers.
- 'Needs assessment' is an important topic for further research. Accurate targeting of resources depends on this task being carried out efficiently and expertly (p. 21).

Notes and references

A more extensive bibliography is available on health promotion and health visiting; see p. xi for details.

1. For two contrasting discussions of child development see Leach, P. (1994). *Children First*. Michael Joseph, London; Burman, E. (1994). *Deconstructing developmental psychology*. Routledge, London.
2. This difficult issue is discussed in Dingwall, R. and Robinson, K. (1993). Policing the family? Health visiting and the public surveillance of private behaviour. In *Health and wellbeing: a reader* (ed. A. Beattie, M. Gott, L. Jones and M. Sidell). Macmillan, Basingstoke.
3. For the contrast with France see Foster, M. (1994). 'Droit de regard au nom de l'état': the juge des enfants and child protection in France. *Children and Society* 8, 200–17.
4. The tasks of health visiting are reviewed in a collection of papers in: Health Visitors' Association (1994). *A power of good: health visiting in the 1990s*. Health Visitors' Association, London.
5. The difficulty in defining need and vulnerability are discussed in Waterfield, J. (1995). Health visiting and children in need. An interim report. (Unpublished, University of East Anglia); Appleton, J.V. (1994). The concept of vulnerability in relation to child protection; health visitors' perceptions. *Journal of Advanced Nursing* 20, 165–75.
6. Health visitors' intuition as a concept was recognized and shown to be valid in a classic study: Neligan, G.A., Prudham, D., and Steiner, H. (1974). *The formative years*. Nuffield Provincial Hospitals Trust/Oxford University Press. A Canadian study investigated how health visitors make decisions: Chalmers, K.I. (1993). Searching for health needs: the work of health visiting. *Journal of Advanced Nursing* 18, 900–11. See also Schon, D. (1983). *The reflective practitioner: how professionals think in action*. Basic Books, New York; Benner, P., Tanner, C., and Chesla, C. (1992). From beginner to expert: gaining a differentiated clinical world in critical care nursing. *Advances in Nursing Science* 14, 13–28.
7. Fonagy, P., Steele, M., Steele, H., Higgitt, A. and Target, M. (1994). The theory and practice of resilience. *Journal of Child Psychology and Psychiatry*, 35, 259–83. (Discusses the important idea that children differ in their ability to cope with adversity.)
8. The concept of 'worthiness' is discussed by Chalmers, K.I. (1993). *Journal of Advanced Nursing* 18, 900–11. Searching for health needs; the work of health visiting. The difficulties of ensuring genuine client participation are described in Kendall, S. (1993). Do health visitors promote client participation? An analysis of the health visitor—client interaction. *Journal of Clinical Nursing* 2, 103–9.
9. Information resources about ethnic issues Hopkins, A. and Bahl, V. (1995). *Access to health care for people from Black and ethnic minorities* Royal College of Physicians, London. See also: Gatrad, A.R. (1994). Atti-

tudes and beliefs of Muslim mothers towards pregnancy and infancy. *Archives of Disease in Childhood* 71, 170–4.

10. Kalnins, I., McQueen, D.V., Backett, K.C., Curtice, L., and Currie, C.E. (1992). Children, empowerment and health promotion: some new directions in research and practice. *Health Promotion International* 7, 53–9.

11. The concept of support is well described in Oakley's studies: e.g. Oakley, A. (1992). *Social support and motherhood*. Blackwell, Oxford.

12. Health promotion in pregnancy is important: see Garcia, J., France-Dawson, M., and Macfarlane, A. (1994). *Improving infant health*. Health Education Authority, London. The Olds study (note 19 below) also implies benefits from establishing a professional relationship during pregnancy.

13. The importance of networks is discussed in social science texts: e.g. Whittaker, J.K., *et al.*, (1983). *Social support networks*. Aldine, New York.

14. Davis, H. and Fallowfield, L. (1991). *Counselling and communication in health care*. J. Wiley, Chichester.

15. The role of paraprofessional staff is addressed in Larner, M., Halpern, R., and Harkavy, O. (1992). *Fair start for children. Lessons learned from seven demonstration projects*. Yale University Press, New Haven, CT. (Of course health care is different in the USA and therefore the situation is not directly comparable with the UK.) See also: Johnson, Z., Howell, F., and Molloy, B. (1993). Community mothers' programme: randomised controlled trial of non-professional intervention in parenting. *British Medical Journal* 306, 1449–52.

16. The topic is reviewed in more detail in Hall, D.M.B. and Hill, P. (1994). Community child health. In *Health care needs assessment* (ed. A. Stevens and J. Raftery), pp. 451–554. Radcliffe Medical Press, Oxford.

17. Chapman, S. (1993). Unravelling gossamer with boxing gloves: problems in explaining the decline in smoking. *British Medical Journal* 307, 429–32. This article takes smoking as an example and explores the influences that determine how and when health education is effective in an individual's life. Recommended!

18. Herbert, E. and Carpenter, B. (1994). Fathers—the secondary partners: professional perceptions and fathers' reflections. *Children and Society* 8, 31–41.

19. The most important study of the potential benefits of health promotion programmes for children is that of Olds, since it used a robust randomized controlled trial design. The results were published in a series of papers. The most recent is Olds, D.L., Henderson, C.R., Jr, and Kitzman, H. (1994). Does prenatal and infancy nurse home visitation have enduring effects on qualities of parental caregiving and child health at 25 to 50 months of life? *Pediatrics* 93, 89–98. For a critique and commentary on Olds' work see Schorr, L.B. (1989). *Within our reach: breaking the cycle of disadvantage*. Anchor Books, New York.

20. Wandersman, L. (1987). Parent–infant support groups: matching programs to needs and strengths of families. In *Research on support for parents and infants in the postnatal period* (ed. C.F.Z. Boudykis), p. 151. Ablex, Norwood, NJ.

21. The importance of poverty as a cause of ill health was highlighted in *Give us a chance: children, poverty and the health of the nation*. Save the Children Fund, London. For a comprehensive literature review up to 1990, see Jolly, D.L. (1990). *The impact of adversity on child health—poverty and disadvantage*. Australian College of Paediatrics, Melbourne. Benzeval, M. Judge K., and Whitehead, M. (1995). *Tackling inequalities in health: an agenda for action*. King's Fund, London.

22. *The book by Larner* et al., (note 15) makes this point very clearly.

23. Profiling relies on a range of local data. See Blackburn, C. (1993). *Poverty profiling*. Health Visitors' Association, London; Reading, R., Openshaw, S., and Jarvis, S. (1994). Are multidimensional social classifications of areas useful in UK health service research? *Journal of Epidemiology and Community Health* **48**, 192–200; Majeed, F.A., Cook, D.G., Poloniecki, J., and Martin, D. (1995). Using data from the 1991 census. *British Medical Journal* **310**, 1511–15.

24. The following deal with specific topics related to targeting: Hodgkin, R. (1994). Government plans for travellers. *Children and Society* **8**, 274–7; Edwards, R. (1992). Coordination, fragmentation, and definitions of need: the new under fives initiative and homeless families. *Children and Society* **6**, 336–52; College of Physicians (1995). *Homelessness and ill health: report of a working party*. Royal College of Physicians, London; Aldridge, J. and Becker, S. (1993). Punishing children for caring: the hidden cost of young carers. *Children and Society* **7**, 376–87; Statham, J. and Cameron, C. (1994). Young children in rural areas: implementing the Children Act. *Children and Society* **8**, 17–30; Kumar, V. (1993). *Poverty and inequality in the UK: the effects on children*. National Children's Bureau, London; Tymchuk, A.J. (1992). Predicting adequacy of parenting by people with mental retardation. *Child Abuse and Neglect* **16**, 165–78.

25. The Audit Commission recommended, as we do, that health visiting should be more targeted: Audit Commission (1994). *Seen but not heard: coordinating community child health and social services for children in need*, para. 118, p. 39. HMSO, London. However, we doubt that the needs of a family previously unknown to the health visitor can be assessed reliably in a single visit.

3
Opportunities for primary prevention

This chapter reviews:
- Immunization and other ways of reducing the incidence of infectious diseases
- Ways of reducing the risk of sudden infant death
- Ways of reducing parental smoking
- Prevention of unintentional injury
- Nutrition and prevention of dental disease
- Situations requiring specialized services

This chapter considers examples of health education interventions aimed at primary prevention.

Reducing the incidence of infectious disease

Increasing triple, polio, and Haemophilus influenza immunization uptake

Although the Working Party did not undertake a detailed review of immunization, the importance of this preventive health care measure is beyond question. However, increasing the uptake is a complex matter.[1] Parents are often confused by the information they receive. The media carry advertising campaigns emphasizing the importance of immunization but also run stories about vaccine damage. Professionals are sometimes ambivalent and ill informed. A firm commitment to immunization among all primary care staff and honest acknowledgment of areas of uncertainty, backed up by an immunization advice service[2], are essential.

An immunization uptake of around 70 or 80 per cent can often be obtained with relatively little difficulty, but considerable professional effort and skill may be needed to ensure that the last 10 or 15 per cent of children are immunized.[3] In a few cases, it may be necessary to immunize a child at home. This can be done by trained nursing staff provided that local protocols have been prepared to ensure that training is adequate and that legal and professional requirements are fulfilled.[4]

Organization is simplified and costs are reduced if, as far as possible, immunizations are carried out on the same occasion as other preventive care activities. Therefore our recommendations (p. 221) take account of the times at which each immunization should be given.

Prevention of tuberculosis

Tuberculosis is still an important problem, particularly among some ethnic groups from areas of high prevalence.[5] The pattern is changing and the incidence appears to be increasing. BCG vaccine should be given to high-risk infants and children, but several local audits suggest that this task is often neglected. When an adult is found to have active pulmonary tuberculosis, contact tracing is mandatory to ensure that any infected child is identified and treated promptly. If this is not done there is a risk, particularly for very young children, that the presenting feature of the illness will be tuberculous meningitis, with potentially devastating consequences.

Hepatitis B vaccine

This is only given to high-risk groups at present, although some authorities believe that it should be universal. The first dose is usually given to neonates in hospital before discharge, but three doses are needed and, as the children involved may be born into families with a variety of other problems, it is easy to overlook the second and third doses (see p. 217).

New vaccines and new programmes

New vaccines may become available in the next few years. An effective vaccine against meningococcal disease is urgently needed. Child health services must be able to respond quickly when a new vaccine or a change in the programme is introduced.

Prevention of other infectious diseases

A variety of strategies could be employed to reduce the risk of infectious diseases among children. Examples include better food and kitchen hygiene, close supervision of young children using toilets in nurseries (where hepatitis and *Shigella* diarrhoea are common problems), and prompt management of outbreaks of meningococcal disease. Parents worry about the risk of toxocariasis leading to blindness. Numerically the risk is very small, but dog fouling of play areas is seen as an important problem by parents. Mothers who are planning a further pregnancy need information about safe eating to reduce risks of listeriosis, toxoplasmosis, etc. The Consultant in Communicable Disease

Table 3.1

The magnitude of the risk of SIDS is related to the following factors:

Social class
Age of mother
Birth interval
Smoking
Infection in pregnancy
Maternal drug addiction
Male infant
Feeding intention (breast or bottle)
Maternal depression
Prematurity or low birth-weight
Multiple births
Congenital defects
Infant sleeping position
Previous sudden infant death

Advice for reducing the risk
This is based on a review carried out by the Foundation for the Study of Infant Deaths (FSID). The three avoidable hazards are as follows:

Parental smoking: parents should not smoke at all; if they cannot give up, they should smoke outside

Overheating: avoid excessive clothing and bedding; bedroom should not be too warm

Sleeping position: baby should sleep supine, or on the side if unable to sleep in this position

Breastfeeding: breastfeeding as a protective factor is of uncertain but probably limited importance. NB Feeding *intention* probably reflects psychosocial factors

Mattresses and covers: recent concerns about toxic gases from mattresses are probably unfounded; loose covers may be hazardous

Control and the Environmental Health Officer are the main sources of expertise on these issues, but primary health care teams should take an active role by providing information and advice for their patients.

Prevention of Sudden Infant Death Syndrome (SIDS) and Sudden Unexpected Death in Infancy (SUDI)[6]

The incidence of SIDS has fallen in recent years and is currently 0.7 per 1000. Some groups of infants are at particular risk of sudden death (Table 3.1). It has been suggested that intensive support and health visiting can reduce this risk. The evidence is inconclusive, but no programme based solely on intervention with high-risk infants will have a major impact on the death rate, since most infant deaths occur in the low-risk group, which numerically is much larger. Therefore the identification of families where more health professional support is required should be based not only on the risk of infant death but also on other broader considerations of need and risk (see p. 33). There is an overlap in the factors which predict an increased risk of child abuse and those which predict sudden death. Many possible reasons have been proposed to explain this association. A minority of sudden deaths are probably non-accidental, but this issue remains controversial.

Some infants who die suddenly have undetectable and irremediable disorders, but others die of potentially treatable conditions. Preventing avoidable deaths involves increased parent awareness of the symptoms and signs of illness in babies. This can be increased by a check list such as Baby Check, although more information is needed on the effectiveness of this tool.[7] Easier access to services and improved professional response to acute illness in babies are also important.

Reduction of smoking by parents

Parental smoking is correlated with a number of adverse outcomes for the child, but it may be difficult to determine whether prenatal or postnatal exposure is the more important factor.[8] A reduction in smoking during pregnancy is a Health of the Nation target.

Children inhale smoke from their parents' cigarettes, so-called passive smoking. Passive smoking has adverse effects on children's health, and there are well-established links between smoking and a variety of adverse outcomes. For example, the risks of SIDS, ear disease, and admission to hospital for respiratory illnesses are significantly increased among the babies of mothers who smoke. Smoking is an important cause of fires in the home. There may also be long-term effects on the risks of adult diseases such as coronary artery disease and cancer.

The effects of passive smoking are not always made sufficiently clear to parents. While it is important not to take a punitive approach, a child's respiratory or ear, nose, and throat illness (pp. 101, 147) offers an ideal opportunity to address the issue. Parents should also be aware of the influence that their smoking may have on their children's smoking behaviour later in childhood.

For many parents smoking is a social activity, a substitute for personal support, and a means of coping with stress. Primary prevention is the ideal solution. Some health professionals feel that it is sometimes insensitive and intrusive to focus on smoking when it is a response to severe life stresses which cannot easily be removed.

Little is known about how best to reduce parental smoking in the first few months of the baby's life. Most research has focused on attempts to reduce smoking in pregnancy. The latter is important, since 90 per cent of women who smoke in pregnancy are still smoking 5 years later. Two-thirds of women who succeed in stopping smoking while pregnant start again after the baby is born. The evidence with respect to fathers' smoking is less clear, but it is probably important at least to the extent that a mother will find it harder to give up smoking if her partner continues.

The aim of reducing smoking should not be pursued in isolation, but rather in the context of more wide-ranging efforts at health promotion within particular families, by creating a good relationship with the parents and promoting self-confidence and self-esteem. Simple advice to stop smoking may not be effective on its own, but when given by a general practitioner it has a significant impact. Support groups, telephone help lines, counselling, and medication may all contribute.

Prevention of unintentional injury

The term 'unintentional injury' is preferred to 'accidents' because the latter implies unpredictability and therefore a negative attitude to the possibility of prevention.[9] Unintentional injuries (including poisonings) are the commonest cause of death and a cause of considerable morbidity in children between the age of 1 and 14 years (Table 3.2). Reducing

Table 3.2 Unintentional injury deaths in children aged 1–4 years, England and Wales 1991*

Motor vehicle accidents, total	67
Motor vehicle accidents, pedestrian	48
Fire and flame	36
Drowning	19
Inhalation and ingestion	15
Falls	8
Suffocation	6
Poisoning	2
Total	170

- Estimated number of injuries in the home in 1989: 647 000.
- Estimated number of poisonings: 40 000 accident and emergency attendances, 14 000 admissions per year.
- Number of children with permanent disability after injury: not known.

*Equivalent statistics for Scotland can be found in *Scottish Accident Statistics 1980–1991*, Report of the Scottish Interdepartmental Working Party on Accidents,

the rate of accidents in children under the age of 15 by 33 per cent by the year 2005 is a Health of the Nation target.

The causes of unintentional injury at different ages reflect the child's state of development, the child's changing perception of danger, and the degree of exposure to different hazards at various ages. Prevention strategies must reflect this and need to address the many different ways in which young children can be injured. Table 3.3 summarizes prevention programmes aimed at reducing the risk of particular types of injury, together with evidence for the effectiveness of the strategies suggested and the implications for prevention programmes.

There is a marked social class gradient, with some injuries being up to six times more common in the poorest areas than in the most prosperous (Table 3.2). Differences in the environment and in social patterns and attitudes underlie this gradient, for example the degree of independence that children are allowed by their parents, the amount of supervision which can be provided on the journey to school, opportunities to play outside the home in safe areas, and differing attitudes to the roles of police, council officers, etc. Where no play facilities exist, young children are often permitted to play in the road outside their home and negotiate road crossings alone before they are old enough to judge the speed of traffic.

Misconceptions abut injuries and accidents

There are many misconceptions about accidents and injuries. For example, parents worry more about the risk of abduction than about road accidents even though the latter are far more common. Although parents are often 'blamed' for accidents and their supposed carelessness is the focus of some prevention strategies, many families, even in the poorest areas, are well aware of potential hazards to their children and know what action they would like to be taken in order to reduce the risk.[10] Similarly, there are myths about the 'accident-prone' child. Although it is true that boys are more likely to have accidents than girls, the majority of children experiencing serious injury are victims of circumstances rather than of their own impulsive actions.

Strategies for prevention

In addition to studies focusing on just one type of injury (Table 3.3), there have been several campaigns aimed at raising awareness of hazards in the home and environment. TV series such as *Play it Safe* are watched by millions of parents. The Newcastle project involved a combination of media coverage with a health-visiting programme in which the messages were tailored specifically to the needs of their target audience. Significant benefits were reported.

At local level, there have been many initiatives such as equipment loan stores (for stair gates, car seats, etc.), first aid courses, swimming lessons, etc. First aid courses may not only help adults to deal with the immediate aftermath of an injury, but also heighten awareness of hazards and thereby reduce the number of injuries.

A campaign in a town in Sweden, involving local policy-makers and the whole community, demonstrated a significant fall in injuries over the study period. The Massachusetts Statewide Child Injury Prevention Campaign (SCIPP) provided five intervention programmes aimed at various types of injury; a significant reduction was shown in only one type (motor vehicle passenger injuries). The difficulties inherent in such campaigns and in demonstrating robust benefits were apparent in this programme:

. . . future interventions must include the active participation of local public health agencies, a media component to increase the awareness of both the public and professionals, and evaluation over a longer time period.[11]

Table 3.3 Injury prevention strategies

Injury type	Implications
MVA—passenger	Children should travel in car seats or restraints. Legislation combined with programmes to promote car safety by loan schemes results in increased use *but* many children still travel without any restraints. **Needs: loan schemes, advertising campaigns, and personal education**
MVA—pedestrian	Educating young children (1–5 age group) unlikely to be effective. Parent education may play a small role—some parents overestimate a young child's capacity for road sense. **Needs: Traffic-calming schemes, traffic-free areas, safe play areas, safer journeys to school.** (NB parents often take their children to school prompted by fear of abduction as well as anxiety about traffic)
Bicycle injuries: horse-riding accidents	Not common in under 5s. Cycle helmet use reduces injury severity. Possibility of rear-pedalling brake for under 5s. **Needs: legislation combined with education.** Few data on horse-riding but importance of safe helmets is recognized
Fire and flame	Burns: house fires important cause. Various causes: smoking, paraffin stoves, electrical and battery fires. Social class gradient—higher risk in inner cities, multiple occupancy, etc. Smoke alarms may reduce morbidity and mortality. If issued free by health authority, need to consider who should receive them, how they are fitted, and how maintained (battery replacement). Other measures, e.g. flame-proofing of nightdresses. Scalds: coiled flexes on kettles, reducing thermostat setting on hot water tanks. **Needs: supply and fitting of smoke alarms (consider as joint responsibility with housing departments).** Check hot water temperature
Drowning	Three main hazards are baths, ponds, and swimming pools. Public swimming bath accidents uncommon. **Needs: parent education about bath dangers*, ponds to be covered, fenced, or drained; swimming pools should be fenced; swimming lessons unlikely to prevent drowning accidents in the preschool age group**

Suffocation* and strangulation	Examples include inhalation of peanuts, sweets etc, plastic bags over the head, being trapped in disused refrigerators, playing games involving 'hanging', etc.
Poisoning	Child-resistant packaging for drugs and medicines—reduced deaths and admissions from poisonings. Still a hazard—some children learn to open ' child-proof' containers. Domestic materials dangers—bleach, paraffin, detergent, paint stripper, etc. **Needs: parent education, continuing improvements in packaging, reminders to parents about potentially lethal toxicity of products that might be thought relatively harmless** (e.g. dishwasher powder, iron tablets, aspirin, children's chemistry sets)
Falls	Falls from high-rise flats (windows and balconies) are potentially fatal. Prevention programmes involve window catches, bars, or guards, making balconies safe, and providing other safer play areas. Playground injuries—risk reduction by use of safer materials and good design. **Needs: collaboration with local authority—housing department and parks/playgrounds; to initiate actions, health visitors need access to carpenter/locksmith/fitter**
Glass injuries (doors, windows, etc.)	Preventable by use of safety glass, membranes, etc. and by good design at planning stage. Little evidence regarding interventions.
Dog attacks	**Needs: parent education about hazards; proper training of dogs; educating children about dog attacks.** Little research available in health sector
Farm accidents	Farm environment is hazardous for young children: animals, machinery, muck heaps, etc.
Sunburn and heat stroke	Severe sunburn in early childhood is risk factor for skin cancer. 'Heat stroke' can occur if children left in cars in full sun. **Needs: parent education**

MVA, motor vehicle accident
* Drowning in baths, especially over the age of 2, and suffocation without clear explanation should be viewed with some suspicion—they may not be accidental

Current status of injury prevention

The prevention of injuries cannot be addressed purely as a health ser-vices issue. Multi-agency planning is essential (Table 3.4). Research findings from other disciplines and agencies, such as the Road Research Laboratory and the Fire Service, must be incorporated into local pol-icy. Health care staff need further information and training in injury prevention.[12] Suitable materials are available though their impact has yet to be fully evaluated.

The inclusion in the personal child health record of a checklist giving examples of hazards and safety checks, based on a developmental per-spective, may enable health professionals to raise the subject with parents more easily. As yet, there is no information as to how effective this might be.

Accident and emergency departments offer an ideal opportunity to monitor accidents and injuries in each district. Information systems should be modified where necessary so that the data required can be obtained easily in an accessible format, allowing local people to have a say in deciding priorities for action. A home visit by a health visitor following an injury may reduce the risk of further accidents, provided that the timing is right and the natural sensitivities of the parents are respected.

Table 3.4   Local accident prevention groups*

There are at least 300 local accident prevention groups

- Some focus only on children, a few only on the elderly and some all age groups
- Accident prevention programmes have been evaluated but there appear to be no formal trials on the impact of local accident prevention groups
- Most groups have concentrated on education and only a few have worked for environmental changes.
- Effective groups are characterized by:
    Adequate resources
    Good relationships and mutual understanding
    Prioritization of tasks
    Intention to achieve specified goals

Accident prevention groups have the potential to be effective but local audit and review should be undertaken

* Information based on the experience of the Child Accident Prevention Trust.

Nutrition

Breastfeeding

Support for breastfeeding is regarded as a priority topic for health promotion.[13] Exclusive breastfeeding until at least 4 and preferably 6 months of age is regarded as the ideal. Breast-fed infants have a reduced risk of infection even in industrialized societies. The protective effect is particularly marked for low birth-weight infants. There may also be other benefits: improved cognitive and psychological development, and reduced risk of juvenile onset diabetes and maternal breast cancer. The evidence regarding protection against allergic disease for those genetically at risk and a reduction in risk of SIDS is more controversial.

The disadvantages of breastfeeding include social limitations (partly determined by societal attitudes and lack of facilities), the uncommon risk of unrecognized underfeeding at the breast, the low levels of vitamin K in breast milk and the association with 'breast milk jaundice', which is a benign condition but may cause anxiety (see p. 135).

In 1980 in England and Wales 67 per cent of women were breast-feeding their babies at the time of discharge from hospital; in 1990 this was marginally reduced to 65 per cent. The figure in Scotland is closer to 50 per cent. When monitoring the level of breast-feeding in a community, it is important to distinguish between intention to breastfeed, initiation, continuation at time of discharge from hospital (if the stay is prolonged), and maintenance. Different strategies are likely to have a differing impact on each of these.

Intention to breastfeed
Women make decisions about breastfeeding early in pregnancy, or even before they become pregnant, influenced by cultural attitudes, social background, and education. There are, therefore, limits to the scope and time-scale for intervention in pregnancy to increase the number of women who intend to breastfeed. Information about the benefits of breastfeeding could be provided in school as part of personal, social, and health education, but very little is known about the effectiveness of this approach.

Establishing lactation
Many women who plan to breast-feed do not persevere in establishing feeding, fail to maintain it after leaving hospital, or give up after a few

Table 3.5   The 'Baby Friendly' initiative

UNICEF will designate a hospital as 'Baby Friendly' if it follows the 10 steps to breastfeeding:

1. Have a written breastfeeding policy routinely communicated to all health staff
2. Train all health staff in skills to implement this policy
3. Inform all pregnant women about the benefits and management of breastfeeding
4. Help mothers initiate breastfeeding within half an hour of birth
5. Show mothers how to breastfeed, and how to maintain lactation, even if they should be separated from their infants
6. Give newborn infants no food or drink other than breast milk, unless *medically* indicated.
7. Practice rooming-in (allow mothers and infants to remain together) 24 hours a day
8. Encourage breastfeeding on demand
9. Give no artificial teats or pacifiers (also called dummies or soothers) to breastfeeding infants
10. Foster the establishment of breastfeeding support groups and refer mothers to them on discharge from the hospital or clinic

---

weeks. Women who intend to breastfeed benefit from positive attitudes and policies in the maternity unit, for example the 'Baby Friendly' initiative (Table 3.5), encouragement and support in problem solving, increased frequency of feeding, discouraging of 'supplementary' feeding, and provision of a breast pump, but no artificial milk, in the free discharge packs offered in maternity units.

Maintenance
Maintenance of breastfeeding is enhanced by lactation counsellors and peer support, which may be more effective than the advice of professionals. The attitude and support of the baby's father are also important factors.

Vitamin K

Current advice about the use of vitamin K is summarized in Table 3.6.

Health information about nutrition

Advice on artificial feeding, weaning, and nutritional supplements is updated regularly in the light of nutritional research,[14] and national

Table 3.6 Vitamin K prophylaxis

- Newborn infants have very low levels of vitamin K which is needed for normal clotting
- Deficiency of vitamin K can lead to haemorrhage at a variety of sites. Bleeding into the brain, though rare, is the most serious. This can occur at any time in the first few months of life. It is important to recognise without delay those babies who are at high risk of bleeding—namely, those with signs of liver disease (see p. 135) or with unexplained bruising.
- Modern formula feeds contain sufficient vitamin K, but babies who are entirely or mainly breast-fed should receive supplements.
- For many years vitamin K was given prophylactically at birth, by intramuscular (i.m.) injection.
- In 1992 a link was suggested between i.m. (but not oral) administration of vitamin K at birth and an increased risk of cancer in childhood.
- The finding has not been confirmed in other studies; nevertheless, it was thought prudent to seek alternative means of prophylaxis, pending the results of further research.
- No one regimen has been shown to be ideal but most involve administration of three doses of oral vitamin K, usually at birth, at 7–10 days and at 28 days. The effectiveness of this approach is still controversial.
- There is currently no licensed oral preparation and many health professionals have been uneasy about taking responsibility for giving oral vitamin K. Various arrangements have been made to overcome this problem.
- There is a risk that the second and third doses, which are usually given after the baby has left hospital, might easily be forgotten, unless the importance of this prophylaxis is stressed to the parents. If serious bleeding were to result, leading to death or permanent disability, the parent might well bring a legal action against the trust concerned.
- There can be no definitive advice on vitamin K prophylaxis until further research results are available. Each district or trust must define its own policy. *If oral preparations are used, a mechanism MUST be in place to ensure that babies of breastfeeding mothers receive ALL the doses specified in the policy, and there must be a means of monitoring the implementation of this policy.*

guidelines are available.[15] These take account of key issues including the prevention of coronary heart disease and obesity, the provision of micronutrients (see also the section on iron deficiency on p. 140) and the hazards of undernutrition.

Specialist advice

Children of vegetarian or vegan parents, and those who need unusual diets for medical reasons, may develop nutritional deficiencies, and specialized advice may be needed from a dietician or nutritionist, who should be familiar with the cultural attitudes of ethnic minority families.[16] Eating disorders and 'failure to thrive' are discussed in the section on weight monitoring (p. 112).

Dental and oral disease

The most common oral diseases in young children—dental caries (tooth decay), periodontal (gum) disease, and dental erosion—are largely preventable.[17]

Dental caries

The main dental disease affecting children, and the one that will probably have the greatest impact on their dental health throughout adult life, is still tooth decay. National and local studies have clearly demonstrated a decline in caries prevalence during the past two to three decades; however, recent surveys reveal a bottoming-out of improvements in the oral health of young children, whilst improvements in older children continue. The decline in 5-year-olds has ceased and local surveys in most parts of the United Kingdom have reported higher decay levels in this age group since 1989.[18]

The national survey of children's dental health in 1993 revealed the following:

- On average, 5-year-old children have two teeth affected by dental caries, and almost half (45 per cent) of this age-group have experienced the disease.

- There is much untreated decay: 40 per cent of 5-year-olds nationally were shown to have active tooth decay.

- Young children who attend the dentist 'only when they had trouble with their teeth' had higher numbers of diseased teeth than those who attended for check-ups, whether every 6 months or less frequently.

- Wide geographical and socio-economic variation in disease levels exists, and there appears to be greater polarization of dental caries experience in 5-year-olds. A greater proportion of this age group have untreated decay.

Nutritional advice

Sugars (non-milk extrinsic sugars) are the most important dietary factor causing dental caries. They are most harmful if eaten or drunk frequently. Prolonged breast- or bottle-feeding beyond the age of 1 year is thought to increase the risk of tooth decay. Good weaning practices contribute to dental health, and parents should be encouraged to wean their children onto food and drink which are, as far as possible, free from non-milk extrinsic sugars.

Fluoride

A level of 1 part per million (ppm) of fluoride in water has been shown to be the most effective method of reducing tooth decay. Although the evidence is compelling, only a minority of the UK population (10–15 per cent) receive fluoridated water. Where it is not available, alternatives include the use of fluoride drops or tablets. Their ingestion is recommended for children at high risk of dental disease from the age of 6 months. Dentists are best placed to identify those individuals who would most benefit from fluoride and to offer it on prescription.

Medicines

Children taking frequent, or regular, sugar-based medicines are known to have increased levels of dental decay. Sugar-containing medicines are still prescribed more frequently by doctors, requested over the counter by parents, and recommended by pharmacists. The use of either solid preparations or sugar-free formulations is preferable for good dental health.

Periodontal (gum) disease

Just over a quarter of 5-year-olds have unhealthy gums due to poor cleaning habits. Effective brushing of teeth and gums using a children's (low-dose) fluoride toothpaste should commence once teeth appear. A small pea-sized blob of paste is all that is required for children up to 6 years of age to prevent unnecessary ingestion of fluoride. Children require parental assistance with brushing until at least 6–7 years of age.

Tooth erosion

Nationally, over half of 5-year-olds have experienced dental erosion: this is the progressive loss of tooth enamel and dentine resulting from chemical action on the teeth, other than that caused by bacteria. This is related to increased consumption of acidic drinks, either as pure fruit juices or as carbonated beverages.

Traumatic damage to teeth

Trauma resulting in loss of or damage to teeth is an important dental problem, best addressed by other measures to reduce unintentional injuries in playgrounds, etc.

Primary prevention strategies

The advice summarized in Table 3.7 should be available to all parents, preferably in the personal child health record, and should be reinforced

Table 3.7   Prevention of dental disease

---

1. Encourage parents in the following practices
    - Avoid the use of sugared dummies and juices in a 'dinky feeder' or night comforter
    - Wean babies onto a diet which, as far as possible, is free from extrinsic non-milk sugars
    - Discourage the use of a bottle after 12 months
    - Restrict the intake of any sugary food and drinks to mealtimes
    - Read labels carefully and beware of 'hidden sugars' in food and drink, even in commercially prepared baby foods
    - Restrict the intake of acidic drinks (carbonated drinks or pure fruit juices) to mealtimes and dilute any fruit juices with water
    - Brush children's teeth, once they appear, using a small toothbrush with a children's fluoride paste (500 ppm fluoride concentration)—no more than a small pea-sized blob of tooth paste is required
    - Commence early and regular dental visits; 6 months of age is the ideal time to seek advice from a dentist on a child's need for fluoride supplements.
    - Encourage dental attendance at least one a year
2. Prescribe and promote the use of sugar-free medicines; when medicines are needed, particularly in the long term, sugary formulations should be avoided; where possible, solid forms or the equivalent sugar-free formulation should be used
3. Refer children with suspected or overt dental disease to a dentist.

---

by staff of the primary health care team. Parents should be reminded that dental advice and treatment, available through the NHS, are free for all children.

Special situations

Some CHP interventions are designed for special groups. Examples include the following:

- CONI (Care of Next Infant)—a programme of support and care for parents who have lost a previous infant through cot death. Though no claims are made that this reduces the risk of the next infant dying, parents value the advice and support they receive.
- Similar support could be offered to parents whose infant has suffered an apparent life-threatening event (previously called near-miss cot death) or to those suffering exceptional anxiety about their infant for other reasons, such as extreme prematurity, oxygen dependency, or tracheostomy.
- Projects to help parents under stress or in need of personal support and development are reviewed on p. 72.
- Assistance in terms of support and developmental guidance to parents of very low birth-weight infants are reviewed on p. 71.
- Specialized advice and guidance for bereaved parents and for parents of children with special needs, i.e. the disabled, the chronically sick and those with life-threatening illness.

Recommendations

- **Immunization rates must continue to be monitored and improvements made wherever possible.** A willingness to immunize at home or during hospital visits and admissions helps to raise uptake rates.
- **The strategy for tuberculosis control should be reviewed.** BCG uptake by eligible children and quality of contact tracing are ideal topics for audit.
- The number of children starting but not completing **hepatitis B** courses should be monitored.
- Health education and prevention strategies for **other infectious dis-**

eases should be reviewed with the consultant in communicable disease control.

- All parents should have access to information about the key points for **reducing the risk of sudden infant death**[18]. This can be included in the personal child health record.

- Services for **parents who need help to stop smoking** should be reviewed and information made available where appropriate. Information about the effect of passive smoking on children should be available.

- Each district should have a multi-agency group to develop and implement a policy for **reducing the risk of unintentional injuries.**

- There should be active support for **breast-feeding** involving hospital maternity units, midwives, health visitors and other professionals. Information about peer group support should be made available.

- A local policy for the use of **vitamin K prophylaxis** should be implemented, formulated, and monitored.

- Since parents are confused by conflicting advice, all health professionals working with children should be familiar with, and base advice on, **national guidelines on nutrition and dental prophylaxis.**

- The PCHT should have access to **specialist advice for children with eating problems** or those who need **unusual diets** for cultural or medical reasons.

- **Information** about CHP should be collected[19] (see p. 215).

Research

Basic research in each of the topics discussed is continuing and will inform future policy. From the CHP perspective, the key issues are how to ensure that the information provided to parents is correct, reliable, and updated regularly, and how best to ensure that the findings of research are translated into acceptable and comprehensible messages for the community as a whole.

Notes and references

A more extensive bibliography is available on health promotion and health visiting; see p. xi for details.

1. Peckham, C.S., Bedford, H.E., Senturia, Y.D., and Ades, A.E. (1989). *The*

National Immunisation Study: factors influencing immunisation uptake in childhood (the Peckham Report). Action Research for the Crippled Child, London. Baxter, D.N. (1994). Pertussis immunisation of children with histories of neurological problems. *British Medical Journal* 309, 1619. Simpson, N., Lenton, S., and Randall, R. (1995). Parental refusal to have children immunised: extent and reasons. *British Medical Journal* 310, 227.

2. Newport M.J., and Conway, S.P. (1993). Experience of a specialist service for advice on childhood immunisation. *Journal of Infection* 26, 295–300.

3. The importance of making additional effort to reach children in deprived situations is highlighted in Reading, R., Colver, A., Openshaw, S., and Jarvis, S. (1994). Do interventions that improve immunisation uptake also reduce social inequalities in uptake? *British Medical Journal* 308, 1142–4.

4. Jefferson, N., Sleight, G., and Macfarlane, A. (1987). Immunisation of children by a nurse without a doctor present. *British Medical Journal* 294, 423–4.

5. Joint Tuberculosis Committee of the British Thoracic Society (1994). Control and prevention of tuberculosis in the United Kingdom; Code of Practice 1994. *Thorax* 49, 1193–1200.

6. Prevention of sudden infant death: for a summary of recent literature, contact The Foundation for the Study of Infant Death, 35 Belgrave Square, London SW1X 8QB (Tel. 0171 235 0965). See also note 18.

7. Morley, C.J., Thornton, A.J., and Cole, T.J. (1991). Baby Check: a scoring system to grade the severity of acute systemic illness in babies under 6 months old. *Archives of Disease in Childhood* 66, 100–5. (Obtainable from the Child Growth Foundation, address on p. 117).

8. Poswillo, D. and Alberman, E. (1992). *Effects of smoking on the fetus, neonate and child*. Oxford University Press, Oxford. (A useful symposium covering the main aspects of smoking and its impact on children's health.) See also *Smoking and pregnancy: guidance for purchasers and providers*, Health Education Authority, London (1994); *Women and smoking*, Guidelines for Health Promotion no. 39. Faculty of Public Health Medicine, London (1995).

9. Two excellent summaries of the literature on injury prevention are (1) Towner, E., Dowswell, T., and Jarvis, S. (1993). *Reducing childhood accidents*. Health Education Authority, London; (2) Avery, J.G., and Jackson, R.H. (1993). *Children and their accidents*. Hodder & Stoughton, Sevenoaks. Two related topics not addressed are sunburn and dogbites. See Marks, R. and Whiteman, D. (1994). Sunburn and melanoma: how strong is the evidence? *British Medical Journal* 308, 75–6; Avner, J. R. and Baker, M.D. (1991). Dog bites in urban children. *Pediatrics* 88, 55–7; Garrett, P. (1991). *Emergency Medicine* 8, 33. See also note 19.
   For advice on prevention of dogbites and dog safety training for children, contact: EarthKind Education Centre (0181 889 1595).

10. Interviews with inhabitants of a deprived housing estate in Scotland showed a high awareness of risks to children: Roberts, H., Smith, S., and

Bryce, C. (1993). Prevention is better . . . . *Sociology of Health and Illness* 15, 447–63.

11. Guyer, B., Gallagher, S., Chang, B., Azzara, C., Cupples, L., and Colton, T. (1989). Prevention of childhood injuries: evaluation of the Statewide Childhood Injury Prevention Program (SCIPP). *American Journal of Public Health* 79, 1521.

12. Health visitors acknowledge the importance of accident prevention but need more training and support: Marsh, P., Kendrick, D., and Williams, E.I. (1995). Health visitors' knowledge, attitudes and practices in childhood accident prevention. *Journal of Public Health Medicine* 17, 193–9.

13. For a comprehensive review of what can be done to improve breastfeeding rates, see Faculty of Public Health Medicine (1995). *Promoting breastfeeding.* Guidelines for Health Promotion, No. 41. Faculty of Public Health Medicine, 4 St Andrew's Place, London NW1 4LB (Tel. 0171 935 0035).

14. Dobbing, J. (1995). *Nestlé Infant Feeding Bibliography.* Available from Nestlé UK Ltd, St George's House, Croydon, Surrey CR9 1NR (Tel. 0181 686 3333).

15. Department of Health (1994). *Weaning and the weaning diet: the COMA report.* HMSO, London.

16. Hall, D.M.B., Hill, P., and Elliman, D. (1994). *Child surveillance handbook*, Radcliffe, Oxford. David, T.J. (1993). *Food and food additive intolerance in childhood.* Blackwell, Oxford.

17. For a summary of the role of preventive dentistry and a list of references, see Sheiham, A. (1994). The future of preventive dentistry. *British Medical Journal* 309, 214–15.

18. Keeley, D. (1995). *Cot death: the tasks for primary health care in prevention and management.* Royal College of General Practitioners, London.

19 Botting, B. (1995). *The health of our children – decennial supplement.* HMSO, London. A statistical overview of many aspects of child health, including accidents, infectious disease etc. – produced by OPCS (Office of Population Censuses and Surveys).

4

Promoting child development

This chapter reviews:
- The aims of CHP with respect to child development
- Ways of helping parents to improve their skills in child care
- Parental mental health
- Language acquisition
- Psychological problems
- Child protection
- Evidence for the effectiveness of primary prevention

Aims

CHP programmes have four aims with respect to child development:

- to promote 'good enough' parenting;
- to reduce the incidence of developmental, emotional and behavioural disorders, parental depression and distress, and child abuse and neglect (primary prevention);
- when this cannot be achieved, to identify disorders as early as possible (secondary prevention);
- to provide support and care for children with permanent disabilities (tertiary prevention).

This chapter reviews the first two of these aims and examines the role of CHP in child development. It addresses the current concerns of parents, and of society as a whole, about the apparently inexorable rise in behavioural problems, educational underachievement, and delinquency among children, and asks what contribution CHP, might make to improving the situation. A separate chapter (Chapter 12) discusses the ways in which disabling conditions can be prevented, identified, and ameliorated.

'Good enough' parenting skills

Bringing up children is not easy. Most parents manage well for most of the time, but for many enjoyment of the task is clouded by uncertainty and lack of information and support. Parents who are confident and consistent in their handling are likely to have more confident and secure children. However, many young people's own experiences of childhood do not offer an ideal model and they may have little opportunity to learn about child development or the maintenance of relationships in families.[1]

Education and preparation for parenthood

There are opportunities for parent training through pre-conceptional and antenatal clinics, and child health services (see box). Although many attempts have been made to provide parent education in a variety of settings, it is often inadequate in quantity and quality, it often excludes fathers (deliberately or otherwise), and it is not always culturally sensitive or acceptable.[2]

Benefits of parent education

... parent support can produce meaningful short-term effects on discrete parenting behaviours; and on parents' efforts at coping, adaptation and personal development. But ... parent support may not set in motion causal processes leading to long term child development outcomes for environmentally at-risk children ... programmes that combine parent support and direct developmental services to young children appear to hold the most promise of promoting improved long-term developmental outcomes, while not neglecting parents' own needs. (Center for Study of Social Policy 1990)

Parent education is defined as:

- A range of educational and supportive measures which help parents and prospective parents to understand their own social, emotional, psychological and physical needs and those of their children and enhances the relationship between them; and which create a supportive network of services within local communities and help families to take advantage of them.
- It consists of three phases:
    Education about parenthood and family life—provided before conception, for example in school.
    Preparation for parenthood—often provided in antenatal classes
    Support for parents—work with parents and child(ren)

(Reproduced with permission from G. Pugh, E. De'Ath, and C. Smith, *Confident parents, confident children*, National Children's Bureau, 1994)

A more substantial investment in personal, social, and health education in the school curriculum might also have benefits, including for example a reduction in the number of teenage pregnancies (a Health of the Nation target).

More research and development is needed in this area and must involve not only health professionals but also social services, schools, and adult education.[3]

The relationship between mothers' mental health and child development

Depression and mood disorders are common among the mothers of young children and occur in all social classes.[4] In low-income deprived populations up to 40 per cent of mothers are depressed and one-sixth have severe psychiatric disturbance.

Maternal depression not only affects the mother's quality of life but also has a number of important implications for the child.[5] The adverse effects include an increased risk of childhood accidents, and an adverse, although complex, impact on behaviour, cognition, and emotional development. Boys are more at risk than girls. The risks of sudden infant death and child abuse may also be increased, although the magnitude of the effect and the mechanism are uncertain. Much less is known about the effect of paternal depression.

The incidence of maternal depression increases threefold immediately after the birth of a baby. Three patterns of postnatal depression are recognized: baby blues (usually transient and self-limiting), which affects 50 per cent of mothers, acute puerperal psychosis, which is rare (1–2 per 1000 births) and needs urgent admission to hospital, and depression with a large reactive component. The first two of these may have a hormonal basis and have little or no relationship with socio-economic status. The third is of particular interest in the present context. About 10 per cent of all mothers are or become depressed within 3 months of giving birth. It is uncertain whether this figure much exceeds that quoted for young women in general, once socio-economic factors have been controlled for.

Prevention of depression

Little is known about primary prevention, but there is some evidence that women at risk can be identified antenatally and that intervention at this stage can reduce the incidence of postnatal depression.

Intervention for depression

It is not always easy to identify postnatal depression. About 50 per cent of cases are missed unless formal enquiries are made. Recognition is facilitated by use of a checklist such as the Edinburgh Postnatal Depression Scale, although it is important to use this with care since to some extent mothers' responses depend on the immediate situation. It is essentially a screening test, and formal psychiatric interview confirms the diagnosis of depression in only about 50 per cent of cases. Very high scores are probably more likely to be significant than borderline scores. Intervention, involving regular visiting and non-directive counselling by health visitors, has been shown in a randomized controlled trial to accelerate recovery, and this encouraging report has been supported by other studies.

Loneliness

Loneliness and isolation are important associates of depression. Although factors such as lack of transport, unfriendly neighbours, and fear of violence play a part, reasons for loneliness lie more in the parents' psychological state—lack of self-confidence, fear of meeting people, and reluctance to accept or reciprocate help. Social isolation is associated with child maltreatment:

People who maltreat children prefer to solve problems on their own. They have few relationships outside the home . . . they tend to be transient, at least in urban areas . . . and to have a lifelong history of avoiding activities that would bring them into contact with other adults . . . . Social isolation does not *cause* maltreatment, but it is an indicator of a lifelong pattern of estrangement[6].

A positive social network will enhance parents' self-image and their perception of family interaction:

Personal networks influence child development in several ways . . . These include the sanctioning of parent behaviour and the provision of material and emotional support for the child. Network members also serve as models for parent and child, they stimulate the child directly . . . these processes stimulate basic trust, empathy and mastery of the skills essential to relationships.[6]

Increasing self-confidence and self-esteem, widening social networks, and initiating new experiences contribute in the long run to improving the parents' health, and this has obvious benefits for the child. The role of health professionals in initiating these changes is discussed on p. 23, and the effectiveness of various programmes aiming to achieve these goals is considered on p. 71.

Promoting language acquisition—looking ahead to school

Concern about speech and language development is a common pre-occupation of parents. Within the health professions, a child who is slow to talk has usually been regarded as if he has a deficit or disorder requiring remediation (see p. 185). There is a great deal of research on *how* children learn to talk, but relatively little has been written from a clinical standpoint about promotion of language acquisition, or primary prevention of disorder and delay,[7] with the obvious exception of identifying hearing defects at an early stage.

A few children have difficulties with speech and language acquisition which are probably determined by genetic or prenatal factors; others are slow because of grossly inadequate care within the home. However, in most cases, neither of these apply.[8] Individual variation in maturation, learning style, and temperament account for much of the difference between children. Variation in the quality of input also affects the rate of language acquisition, and the same applies to play (see box). The extent to which these insights can or should be applied when advising parents is still an open question, but carefully controlled manipulation of child–adult interactions might accelerate development in some circumstances. Structured communication groups in day nurseries also produce measurable benefits in language and in other areas of development.[9]

What are the relative contributions of child and adult to the process of language learning? The answer must be stated in terms of an interaction. Interaction, first, between the child's predisposition to learn to communicate and the model of language provided by those who communicate with him. Interaction, also, in the form of the specific conversations that provide the evidence from which the child learns and feedback on how his own communications are interpreted by others.

In the course of development, each child reconstructs language afresh from the evidence that is made available to him or her. Yet, because of the similarity between children in the resources and strategies they bring to bear on this task, there is considerable uniformity in the sequence in which it is achieved. Nevertheless, to recognize the child's active involvement is not to deny the important contribution of parents and other caretakers. They provide the conversational scaffolding within which this construction takes place. Nor is it to ignore the differences that exist between adults in their ability or willingness to fulfil this role . . . . There is clearly observable variation in the quality and quantity of the conversational experience that children enjoy with adults and this is associated with differences in the ease and speed of their language development. Some parents more than others appear intuitively to know how to facilitate their children's learning.

Those whose children are most successful are not concerned to give systematic linguistic instruction but rather to ensure that conversations with their children are mutually rewarding. They assume that, when their child speaks, he or she has something to communicate, so they try to work out what it is and, whenever possible, to provide a response that is meaningful and relevant to the child and that invites a further contribution. By employing strategies that enable their children to participate more fully and successfully in conversation, these parents sustain their children's motivation to communicate and this, in turn, increases their opportunities to discover the means for realizing their communicative intentions more effectively.

The facilitation is not all in one direction, however. The children themselves differ in their willingness to engage in interaction and, at each stage, in the meanings and purposes that they most frequently attempt to communicate. The source of these individual differences is still to be discovered, but they, too, contribute to the forms that particular conversations take and perhaps also to the process of language learning. Thus, whilst the adult, as the more mature communicator, has the major responsibility for sustaining and extending the child's conversational contributions, this can only be achieved within the parameters set by the child's own individual interests and inclinations. In this sense too, therefore, language learning takes place through interaction.

Reproduced with permission from: Wells, G. (1985). *Language development in the pre-school years*. Cambridge University Press, Cambridge.

There is a natural continuity from spoken language acquisition to reading and writing, and this is recognized in the National Curriculum for English, which has three Profile Components—Speaking and Listening, Reading, and Writing. So far, there has been little research on how the natural concerns of parents about spoken language and reading skills could be linked together.[10] There is evidence that developing 'phonological awareness' by rhyming games, for example, may help reading. A number of other activities may also be useful. Learning to listen, attend, and use learning strategies are important skills to acquire before starting school.[11] Perhaps the most important barrier to be overcome is the reluctance of professionals to 'trust' parents to be more involved in teaching their children.[12]

Primary prevention of behavioural and psychological problems

The incidence of emotional and behavioural difficulties (EBD) in schools is currently a matter of great concern.[13] The pressures on schools resulting from recent educational reforms may result in a greater willingness to label children as EBD. Placement in a special school or exclusion from school may result.[14] Children designated EBD are likely to have experienced some or all of the following: lack of parental interest in schooling, inconsistent and ineffectual discipline, lack of overt parental affection, parental hostility or rejection, violent displays of temper, corporal punishment, cruelty or neglect, and parental absences. Not surprisingly, there is some overlap between these factors and those associated with overt child abuse.

What little is known about prevention of these problems suggests that primary prevention programmes have not been very successful.[15] An 'inoculation' model (e.g. early short-term education for parents) appears to be less useful than a 'nutritional' model which provides input throughout childhood in 'doses'. If this is correct, then sustained professional contact would be important, as was found in Olds' studies (see note 19, p. 39).

Improving attachment behaviour

Insecure infant–parent attachment is an important predictor of social and emotional problems in later childhood and adult life, and may lead to similar problems in the next generation. One key factor is the sensitivity of the parent to the infant's attachment signals. There is some evidence that parents who have difficulties in managing their infants can be helped to respond more effectively, and that this might have long-term benefits.[16]

Liaison with education professionals

Some antecedents of difficult behaviour can be observed even in preschool children. Collaboration is needed between health and educational professionals if early intervention to prevent behavioural problems in the pre-school years is to be continued successfully in primary school.

Somatizers

There is some evidence that adults who respond to life stresses by exhibiting physical symptoms—the so-called somatizers—learn this pattern of response in childhood, and there may be scope for primary prevention, by recognizing this at an early stage and helping parent and child to find more positive ways of coping with stress. The benefits of successful prevention would be considerable for both the individual and the health service; in addition, there might be beneficial effects on school attendance.[17]

Child protection—prevention of child abuse and neglect

Child abuse is a common and important problem. In 1993 there were 42 600 initial child protection case conferences in England and 32 500 children were on local authority child protection registers* (a rate of 29.6 per 1000). Of these, 26 per cent were for neglect, 37 per cent for physical injury, 26 per cent for sexual abuse, 11 per cent for emotional abuse, and 8 per cent for grave concern (a category now withdrawn).[18]

There have been many studies of the risk factors which predict an increased likelihood of child abuse.[19] Reduction in the risk of child abuse and neglect is one of the outcome measures used in research studies of home visitation and health visiting (see below). The distinction between primary and secondary prevention is rather blurred in dealing with child protection issues. There is some evidence that primary prevention can be achieved in high-risk families, characterized by single-teenager parenthood and poverty; it is as yet inconclusive for other situations.[20]

The causes and antecedents of child maltreatment are complex. The

* In Scotland, there were 2677 children on child protection registers at the end of March 1993.

Table 4.1 Examples of risk factors for child abuse[19] (after Browne)

---

1. History of family violence
2. Parent indifferent, intolerant, or overanxious towards child
3. Single or separated parent
4. Socio-economic problems such as unemployment
5. History of mental illness, drug or alcohol addiction
6. Parent abused or neglected as child
7. Infant premature, low birth-weight
8. Infant separated from mother for more than 24 hours postdelivery
9. Mother less than 21 years old at the time of birth
10. Step-parent or cohabitee present
11. Less than 18 months between birth of children
12. Infant mentally or physically handicapped

---

truly psychopathic or mentally ill abuser is relatively uncommon. More often, abuse occurs as a result of multiple factors involving the child, the parents, their life situation, and a series of events which lead to abuse, the so-called 'critical path'. With increasing understanding of child abuse, lists of 'risk factors' have been developed (Table 4.1) but, although these enable a high-risk population to be identified, this 'screening' approach is not sufficiently sensitive or specific to be used as a means of allocating resources to individual families. Nevertheless there is an overlap with the list of indicators which might be used by health visitors when assessing needs for health care in a more general sense (p. 33).

Prevention of child abuse in the majority of families is just one of the aims of a CHP programme. Parents are very aware of child abuse issues and would expect to be told if their health visitor or another professional had concerns about the care of their child. In most instances, honesty is far preferable to a secretive approach. Topics such as the often unrecognized hazards of shaking a baby provide a non-threatening and non-stigmatizing way of introducing the subject in all families and not just in those designated as 'high risk'. A leaflet on this theme has recently been produced and can be adapted for use in the personal child health record (but see p. 25).

Failure to thrive

The problems of identifying failure to thrive as a marker of neglect or abuse are discussed on p. 112.

Child sexual abuse

Education programmes for children, aimed at the primary prevention of child sexual abuse and abduction, are effective under experimental conditions, but their impact in real-life situations is not yet established. Little is known about ways of preventing young people and adults from becoming perpetrators. Responsibility for preventing sexual abuse should not be placed solely on children.

Female genital mutilation

Recently there has been concern about female genital mutilation among immigrant groups in the UK.[21] This is a traditional practice in various cultures, mainly of African origin. There are many types of procedure, but the more extensive ones are the cause of much pain, disfigurement, and distress. These procedures are illegal in the UK but prevention requires considerable tact, diplomacy, and insight into the customs and cultures concerned.

Secondary prevention

Secondary prevention is the focus of much child protection work. It involves early recognition of warning signs and appropriate action, as dictated by local and national guidelines. Tertiary prevention such as victim and family counselling may also be important.

Working with social services

The importance of close liaison between health care professionals, social services, and education authorities is emphasized in the Children Act. Areas where collaboration is particularly vital include child protection and children with disabilities. There is a legal requirement that children Looked After by the local authority should have a medical assessment every 6 months under the age of 2 and annually thereafter (unless the child is of an age and understanding to refuse). Local policy must specify how these obligations are to be discharged.

What evidence of effectiveness is available?

Several studies (see box) indicate the potential benefit of intensive early intervention programmes designed to promote child development, improve parents' mental health and self-esteem, and reduce the risks of child abuse and accidental injury. The *characteristics* of successful programmes are summarized on p. 31.

However, there is no room for complacency. Little is known of the overall impact on child abuse of our current identification and management procedures and even less about their cost-effectiveness.

Examples of intervention programmes
Programmes subjected to randomized trials
The impact of intensive health-visiting programmes The best documented study is the one conducted by Olds in the USA. Intensive home visiting by trained nurses (equivalent to UK health visiting but with a much smaller case load), when targeted to poor unsupported teenage mothers, improved obstetric outcomes, reduced hospital admissions and child abuse (for the duration of the programme), and had a positive impact on the development, behaviour, home safety, and injury rates. The benefits were marginal when home visiting was undertaken for more prosperous women. The effectiveness of the programme was said to decline as soon as the level of funding and professional support was reduced.[22]

The impact of structured home-visiting programmes using non-qualified or paraprofessional staff In general, these have been less intensive and less ambitious in their aims. In a series of studies with populations of poor and deprived families in the USA, supported by the Ford Foundation (Child Survival/Fair Start) the measurable benefits included better utilization of health care facilities, including immunization uptake; however, these may reflect the greater difficulty in accessing the health care system in the USA. There were small improvements in developmental scores, but little impact was found on smoking behaviour, uptake and maintenance of breast-feeding, weaning practices, or birth outcomes.[23]

The long-term outcomes of early intervention delivered primarily in the educational sector High quality 'compensatory education' for the children of poor families does not increase IQ, but it does have other long term benefits. These include higher achievements in school and in the job market, and reduced rates of crime and marital breakdown. In contrast, day nursery provision, where structured approaches to learning cannot so readily be provided, may meet a social need but does little to change either immediate developmental progress or long term outcomes.[24]

Benefits of early intervention for low birth-weight infants The Infant Health and Development Program was a randomised trial of a 36 month intensive developmental intervention programme for infants of very low birth weight (<1500gm). Cognitive development scores in the intervention group were 9.4 points higher after excluding those with overt brain damage (cerebral palsy). Infants weighing <1000gm at birth had lower behaviour problem scores. The benefits were mainly seen in the infants of mothers of low socio-economic status and little advantage was seen in children of better educated mothers.[25] Other reports also indicate that such targetted interventions might be beneficial.[26]

Programmes for which mainly descriptive reports are available
The Bristol Child Development Programme involves approximately 20 000 UK families each year. There are several programme models, including the First Parent Visiting Programme, the Integrated Urban and Rural Models, and the Community Mothers Programme. The programmes are based on monthly home visits to families, either by health visitors or by experienced mothers drawn from local communities[23]. Key features include a strong emphasis on empowering parents to find their own solutions to their child-rearing concerns rather than advising them how to do so, a semi-structured approach with a behavioural emphasis and the provision of information through light-hearted cartoon material. Various evaluation studies have been undertaken during the past 15 years. It is claimed that benefits can be demonstrated in all of these measures but a full evaluation has not yet been published. Further information can be obtained from the Early Childhood Development Unit, University of Bristol, 22 Berkeley Square, Bristol BS8 1HP, UK.

45 Cope Street (an example of a local project to support parents) is a preventative health care service which works in partnership with young pregnant women and young mothers (16–25 years) and their children. The aim is to improve child and family health, and to develop the client's parenting skills through group work and involvement in the creche. Client and worker evaluation has always been an inbuilt part of the work at 45 Cope Street in order to monitor and improve the service. A report consolidating this evaluation was published in 1991 and can be obtained from 45 Cope Street, Hyson Green, Nottingham, NG7 5AB, UK.

Homestart was founded in 1973. It is a large voluntary organization in which volunteers offer regular support, friendship, and practical help to young families under stress in their own homes, helping to prevent family crisis and breakdown. Each local scheme is independent and has a paid organizer who recruits volunteers and visits families referred to the scheme to assess their needs. Volunteers are usually mothers themselves and aim to befriend families who are having difficulties, reassure and support them, and help them to make friends and use services more effectively. Homestart complements the statutory services and aims to reduce the need for professional intervention. A detailed description has been published but no formal evaluation has been made. Further information can be obtained from Homestart, 2 Salisbury Road, Leicester LE1 7QR, UK. (tel. 0116 255 4988: fax 0116 254 9323.

Newpin (New Parent Infant Network) is a large voluntary organization in the UK providing help for people with parenting difficulties. It was established in 1980 with the aim of preventing family breakdown. There are currently ten centres in England providing a 'package' of social involvement, therapy, and training. People are referred to Newpin by a wide range of agencies, or may self-refer. The 'Newpin process' begins with a home visit by a centre coordinator. If Newpin is thought to be appropriate, the next step is attachment to a centre via being 'matched' with a volunteer befriender already involved in Newpin. Centres provide a drop-in and a creche. Training programmes include a personal development programme (PDP), which uses therapy to explore the personal roots of parenting difficulty and to promote self-esteem. Newpin emphasizes the value of a caring community based on a non-hierarchical model of support in which those who have been helped then go on to help others. Evaluations indicate some benefits for some of the women, but changes in the children have been difficult to demonstrate. Further information can be obtained from National Newpin, Sutherland House, 35 Sutherland Square, London SE17 3EE, UK (tel. 0171 703 6326: fax 0171 703 2660).

Portage The Portage home teaching scheme was developed in the Portage area, Wisconsin, USA, in the early 1970s to meet the needs of young children living in rural communities. Portage is a home-visiting educational service for preschool children who have special needs. It is based on the common-sense principle that parents are the key figures in the care and development of their child. Portage assesses the needs of young children with learning difficulties, including those with physical disabilities, and then, in partnership with parents, builds on the abilities that the child already has, teaching skills that the child has yet to master. A Portage team of home visitors offers a carefully structured but flexible system to help parents become effective teachers of their own children. Portage aims to help parents continue to gain satisfaction and success in their role as the main influence of their child's development. With Portage, the parent–child link is consolidated and enriched. Portage materials and handbook are available from: NFER-Nelson, Darville House, 2 Oxford Road East, Windsor, Berkshire 5L4 1DF (tel. 01753 858961: fax 01753 856830).

Conclusion

It is difficult at present to make firm recommendations. There is ample evidence that much more could be accomplished, but so far the evidence is based mainly on demonstration projects and research programmes, which are usually better staffed and supported than routine service work.

Primary prevention of developmental problems and child abuse can be achieved at least to some extent, but there is probably a level of service below which no benefits will be discernible. It follows that an intensive service (such as envisaged in the Bristol or Olds' programmes), when targeted to carefully selected individuals who are fully engaged with the professional effort, may be useful and cost-effective, but a low-intensity service provided to large numbers of parents is less likely to be useful.

Recommendations

- Districts should consider how best to provide an intensive support service **targeted to a carefully defined and selected population** and aimed at improving behavioural, developmental, and nutritional outcomes, and reducing the risk of neglect and abuse.
- This should be undertaken, initially on a pilot basis, in **partnership with education authorities, social services, and voluntary organizations.**
- A philosophy of true **parent–professional partnership** is essential.
- In order to make this possible, the **optimum use of resources** will need to be considered.

Research

- Further work is needed on how best to apply the insights of basic research in developmental psychology, language, early education, etc. in the 'real world' and how to monitor the benefits.

Notes and references

A more extensive bibliography is available on health promotion and health visiting; see p. xi for details.

1. Pugh, G., De'Ath, E., and Smith, C. (1994). *Confident parents, confident children.* National Children's Bureau, London. (This book reviews the literature on parenting and has extensive references.)
2. Combes, G. and Schonveld, A. (1992). *Life will never be the same again.* Health Education Authority, London. (An excellent review of the potential for antenatal parent education: useful bibliography). Also obtain the

companion book: Braun, D. and Schonveld, A. (1993). *Approaching parenthood: a resource for parent education.* Health Education Authority, London.

3. Adcock, M., and White, R. (1994). *Good enough parenting.* British Association for Adoption and Fostering, London. (For recognition of parenting problems, see in particular the chapter by Cooper.)

4. Postnatal depression is a complex subject. Some authors have addressed it as a social phenomenon, and others as a medical problem. For an overview, see Cox, J. and Holden, J. (ed.) (199?). *Perinatal psychiatry.* Gaskell/Royal College of Psychiatrists, London. The sociological perspective is reviewed in Sheppard, M. (1994). Postnatal depression, child care and social support: a review of findings and their implications for practice. *Social Work and Social Sciences* 5, 24–46.

5. There is persuasive evidence (a) that early intervention results in a more rapid improvement in postnatal depression ratings and (b) there is an association between postnatal depression and various developmental measures. It is logical to suppose that early intervention will benefit the child but the existence and magnitude of this effect have yet to be fully evaluated.

6. Whittaker, J.K., *et al.* (1983). *Social support networks.* Aldine, New York (p. 183; 177–8).

7. See notes and references on pp. 209–11.

8. Pinker, S. (1994). *The language instinct.* Allen Lane/Penguin Press, London. (A state of the art review on language acquisition—essential reading.)

9. Best, W., Melvin, D., and Williams, S. (1993). The effectiveness of communication groups in day nurseries. *European Journal of Disorders of Communication* 28, 187–212. (A randomized controlled trial showing significant benefits of intervention groups in language and other preschool skills.)

10. Hannon, P. (1995). *Literacy, home and school.* Falmer Press, London. (An up-to-date review of reading and pre-reading skills, including a focus on what parents can do to help.)

11. Wells, G. (1985). *Language development in the pre-school years.* Cambridge University Press.

12. Concern about deprivation is natural but the creation of opportunities for gifted children should not be forgotten. See Freeman, J. (1995). Recent studies of giftedness in children. *Journal of Child Psychology and Psychiatry* 36, 531–48.

13. Farrell, P. (1995). *Children with emotional and behavioural difficulties.* Falmer Press, London.

14. Parents are increasingly concerned about exclusions from school: see Blyth, E. and Milner, J. (1993). Exclusion from school: a first step in exclusion from society? *Children and Society* 7, 255–68.

15. See notes and references on p. 209–11.

16. Rutter, M. (1995). Clinical implications of attachment concepts: retrospect and prospect. *Journal of Child Psychology and Psychiatry* 36, 549–72.

17. This paragraph is somewhat speculative, but the topic is worthy of further study. See Whitehead, W.E., Crowell, M.D., Heller, B.R., Robinson, J.C., Schuster, M.N., and Horn, S. (1994). Modelling and reinforcement of the sick note during childhood predicts adult illness behaviour. *Psychosomatic Medicine* **56**, 541–50.
18. An annual statistical review is available from the Department of Health: *Children and young people on child protection registers.*
19. For example Browne, K. (1995). Preventing child maltreatment through community nursing. *Journal of Advanced Nursing* **21**, 57–63. Browne, K. (1995). Predicting maltreatment. *In* P. Reder (Ed.), *Assessment of parenting,* J. Wiley, Chichester, pp. 118–35. Browne describes the risk factors but emphasizes that there are no easy solutions to screening, assessment, or intervention. Burrell, B., Thompson, B., and Sexton, D. (1994). Predicting child abuse potential across family types. *Child Abuse and Neglect* **18**, 1039–49.
    The case against individual risk scoring approaches is argued by Baldwin, N. and Spencer, N. (1993). Deprivation and child abuse: implications for strategic planning in children's services. *Children and Society* **7**, 357–75.
20. For authoritative reviews of the literature on primary prevention of child abuse and maltreatment, see MacMillan, H.L., MacMillan, J.H., Offord, D.R., Griffith, L. and MacMillan, A. (1994). Primary prevention of child physical abuse and neglect: a critical review: parts I and II, *Journal of Child Psychology and Psychiatry* **35**, 835–56, 857–76. For an overview of how child protection can be evaluated see: Thorpe, D. (1994). *Evaluating child protection.* Open University Press, Buckingham.
21. Toubia, N. (1994). Female circumcision as a public health issue. *New England Journal of Medicine* **331**, 712–6.
    Webb, E. and Hartley, B. (1994). Female genital mutilation: a dilemma in child protection. *Archives of Disease in Childhood* **70**, 441–4.
22. See note 19 on p. 39.
23. See note 15 on p. 39. For an account of an innovative approach in Dublin, see Johnson, Z., Howell, F., and Molloy, B. (1993). Community Mothers' programme: randomised controlled trial of non-professional intervention in parenting. *British Medical Journal* **306**, 1449–52.
24. Ball, C. (1994). *Start right: the importance of early learning.* Royal Society of Arts, London. (Argues the case for early educational input for all children; extensive bibliography.)
25. McCormick, M.C., McCarton, C., Tonascia, J., and Brooks-Gunn, J. (1993). Early educational intervention for very low birth weight infants: results from the Infant Health and Development Program. *Journal of Pediatrics* **123**, 527–33.
26. Wolke, D. (1991). Supporting the development of low birthweight infants. *Journal of Child Psychology and Psychiatry* **32**, 723–41.

5

Secondary prevention: early detection and the role of screening

This chapter:
- Asks whether early detection matters
- Asks how early detection can be achieved
- Considers the role of professional help in the early detection of problems
- Introduces the topic of screening
- Comments on the need for professional sensitivity
- Defines screening
- Sets out the criteria for screening programmes and screening tests
- Describes and explains recent changes in attitudes to screening.
- Explains how the Working Party attempted to evaluate existing screening programmes

Inevitably, much of this report focuses on the question of early detection. In particular, screening programmes generate fierce controversies and there are wide variation in standards of practice. Nevertheless, we wish to emphasize again that the detection of defects is only one of the aims of a CHP programme and is by no means the most important.

Does early detection matter

The Working Party considered first whether early detection is a legitimate goal for a CHP service. It is not possible to give a precise definition of 'early', but the word implies that defects should be found at the earliest stage of the disease or disability that is reasonably possible, rather than waiting until they are inescapably obvious. We believe that early detection is desirable on a number of grounds.

Parents value early diagnosis

The most compelling reason for early diagnosis is that parents want it. We identified both research evidence and a weight of clinical opinion in favour of this view. Parents feel that they have a right to know of any concerns about a child's development at the earliest possible stage. Early diagnosis, if accompanied by adequate counselling, facilitates adaptation and adjustment to the problems created by disability, even when the underlying disorder is not amenable to specific treatment.

It is interesting to consider why parents should value early detection so highly, even when it does not result in any effective treatment or in relevant genetic counselling. The reason is probably to do with the 'loss of the perfect child' which is distressing when a serious defect is discovered at birth, but is even more so as the child grows older; the longer the parents believe him to be normal, the more devastating is the discovery that he is not.

Improved outcome

In a few disorders, there is no doubt that detection and treatment at the presymptomatic stage improve outcome. Examples include phenylketonuria and hypothyroidism. There are also disorders where it is probable that early detection and treatment improve outcome, but the evidence is equivocal. A good example is congenital sensorineural hearing loss. Sometimes early diagnosis has no direct effect on the child but permits genetic counselling which may prevent the birth of another child with the same disorder. An example is Duchenne muscular dystrophy.

Improved quality of life for child and family

There are many disorders in which early identification does not improve outcome in the sense of significantly altering the severity of the disability. Nevertheless, appropriate intervention enables the child and family to cope with disability more effectively by reducing parental frustration and isolation, providing services, and helping the child to make the most effective use of any functions and abilities that are preserved. For example, in the case of cerebral palsy, early physiotherapy can prevent or delay the progression of postural deformities and contractures.

Access to Educational and Social Services

Education authorities need to know about children with special needs in order to offer preschool teaching[1] and to enable them to fulfil their responsibilities under the Education Act 1993. Similarly, social services have certain obligations under the Children Act 1989. Furthermore, parents may be entitled to financial benefits in some situations.

No legal duty has been imposed on health authorities or trusts to *detect* children with special needs. However, there is a legal requirement to inform the local education authority 'when they form the opinion that a child under 5 may have special educational needs and they must also inform the parents if they believe that a particular voluntary organization is likely to be able to give the parent advice or assistance in connection with any special educational needs that the child may have' (1994 Code of Practice, Section 176).[2]

How early detection is achieved

A large proportion of serious problems are found in one of five ways:

- the neonatal and 6–8 week examinations;
- follow-up of infants and children who have suffered various forms of trauma or illness affecting the nervous system;
- detection by parents and relatives
- detection by midwives, playgroup leaders, nursery nurses and teachers, health visitors, and general practitioners in the course of their regular work;
- opportunistic screening.

Neonatal and 6–8 week examinations

The neonatal examination and the examination performed at around 6–8 weeks of age reveal a significant number of abnormalities, for example dysmorphic conditions such as Down's syndrome, congenital heart disease, and anomalies of the eyes.

Neurological illnesses

Infants who have suffered illnesses or insults with the potential to cause neurological damage are normally seen regularly in a specialist clinic. A significant proportion of the severely disabled children known to any child development team are recognized by a paediatrician as being actually or potentially disabled as soon as the neurological insult occurs. Examples include premature infants whose imaging studies show persisting brain abnormalities, babies who have suffered hypoxic-ischaemic encephalopathy, neonatal meningitis, or severe hypoglycemia, and infants and children who have had meningitis, encephalitis, head injury, or encephalopathy. Thus many of the disabled infants in any district can be identified and offered early intervention if a well-organized follow-up clinic is available.

We are not advocating a return to the concept of an 'at-risk' register by which risk factors are recorded with a view to alerting community staff to the possibility of developmental problems.[3] This approach to detection of defects was introduced at a time when (i) resources were very limited and (ii) undue emphasis was placed on perinatal factors in the aetiology of developmental disorders and defects. It fell into disrepute for two reasons: firstly, it was impossible to obtain consistent reporting and recording of the relevant risk factors; secondly, many children found to have serious disabling conditions had no antecedent risk factors.

The role of parents and relatives

Parents, sometimes with the aid of relatives and friends, are often the first to recognize that their child has a disability. They use their own knowledge, based on experience, television, radio, books, and magazines, and make comparisons with the babies of their friends and relatives before deciding that their child may not be developing normally. When they report these suspicions to a health professional they often prove to be correct.

The parents are often the first to recognize visual impairment, cerebral palsy, muscular dystrophy, severe learning disability, sensorineural deafness, and autism. They may not understand the significance of their observations but they are very efficient at detecting that something is amiss. When anxious parents seek help, they must receive a sympathetic hearing. It is vital that all staff respect and respond to parental worries.

Playgroup leaders, nursery nurses, and nursery teachers

These play an increasingly important role in child care, particularly in deprived areas. They become expert at recognizing the child whose health or development require further evaluation. The value of their contribution should be recognized.

Opportunistic detection

Some defects and conditions are first suspected in the course of a consultation or contact arranged for some other reason. This might be described as 'opportunistic detection'.

All parents need help sometimes—the role of professional advice

Parents have the key role in the detection of defects, but they seldom decide instantaneously that their child might have some abnormality of health or development. The conclusion is reached gradually after discussion and observation. Nor do they always know how to make the best use of health, educational, or social services.

Formation of a constructive relationship between professional and family has several benefits. Firstly, it facilitates primary prevention by providing guidance on health and development. Secondly, such a relationship makes it easier for the parents to seek advice when they have anxieties about their child. Contact with a professional who has a knowledge of child development enables them to clarify and crystallize their worries and to decide whether and when they wish to obtain more expert advice. Such decisions are not taken lightly. Although most parents are grateful for assessment and support, they are also very anxious about what the outcome will be.

Therefore a routine review of the child's progress can be valuable in some circumstances, even if the parents have not sought advice or expressed concerns. It also helps them to observe their child's progress more objectively and to identify possible problems themselves.

For a variety of reasons parents sometimes fail to recognize, or understand the significance of, symptoms of illness or developmental abnormalities which might seem obvious to other people. The reasons for their lack of awareness are often complex and are not related solely to social background or education. Parents may seek to rationalize their observations of problems such as slow language development on many grounds, for example normal variation, unusual family history, or adverse life experiences. The opportunity to review these problems

without having to request a formal appointment may be much appreciated. Professionals should invite parents' views before expressing their
own opinion.

The role of formal screening programmes

Some defects are unlikely to be recognized even by the most astute parent
and can only be detected by health professionals if a specific search is
made. Examples include congenital dislocation of the hip before the
child starts to walk, high-frequency hearing loss before the age when
speech normally begins, and some inherited metabolic disorders. The
detection of such defects might be achieved by the use of specific
screening tests. This is discussed below.

The need for professional sensitivity

When a problem has been overlooked by parents, its identification by
professionals during screening or routine reviews is often welcomed.
There may also be less positive responses, though these may be con-
cealed. Parents may have been actively denying the possibility of there
being anything wrong with the child to protect themselves or their
partners against a distressing experience; this may happen particularly
at times when they are having to deal with several other sources of
stress and anxiety. Alternatively, parents may feel guilt that they had
failed to identify the problem or act upon it until it was pointed out to
them.

   These phenomena are not a reason for withholding information
or failing to be honest about one's suspicions, but they do highlight
the need for professional skill, sensitivity, and follow-up support and
guidance when carrying out child health checks.

Screening

Definition

Screening was defined by the American Commission on Chronic Illness
in 1957 as 'the presumptive identification of unrecognized disease or
defect by the application of tests, examinations and other procedures,

which can be applied rapidly. Screening tests sort out apparently well persons who may have a disease from those who probably do not. A screening test is not intended to be diagnostic'.

Criteria for screening programmes and tests

The concept of screening is attractive.[4] It makes good sense to identify disease or disorder at a presymptomatic stage in order to correct it before too much damage is done. Recognizing that the number of diseases for which screening might in theory be possible is almost unlimited, Wilson and Jungner[5] devised a set of criteria by which screening programmes could be evaluated (Table 5.1).

Table 5.1 Wilson and Jungner's criteria for screening programmes

1. The condition to be sought should be an important public health problem *as judged by the potential for health gain achievable by early diagnosis*

2. There should be an accepted treatment *or other beneficial intervention for* patients with recognized *or occult* disease

3. Facilities for diagnosis and treatment should be available *and shown to be working effectively for classic cases of the condition in question*

4. There should be a latent or early symptomatic stage *and the extent to which this can be recognized by parents and professionals should be known*

5. There should be a suitable test or examination: it should be simple, valid for the condition in question, reasonably priced, repeatable in different trials or circumstances, sensitive and specific; the test should be acceptable to *the majority of* the population

6. The natural history of the condition *and of conditions which may mimic it* should be understood

7. There should be an agreed definition of what is meant by a case of the target disorder, and *also an agreement as to (i) which other conditions are likely to be detected by the screening programme and (ii) whether their detection will be an advantage or a disadvantage*

8. Treatment at the early, latent, or presymptomatic phase should favourably influence prognosis, *or improve outcome for the family as a whole*

9. The cost of screening should be economically balanced in relation to expenditure on the care and treatment of persons with the disorder and to medical care as a whole

10. Case finding *may need to be* a continuous process and not a once and for all project, *but there should be explicit justification for repeated screening procedures or stages*

Modifications proposed to increase relevance for paediatric practice are shown in italics.

Cochrane and Holland described the characteristics of the ideal screening test as follows:

1. Simple, quick, and easy to interpret: capable of being performed by paramedics or other personnel.
2. Acceptable to the public, since participation in screening programmes is voluntary.
3. Accurate, i.e. gives a true measurement of the attribute under investigation.
4. Repeatable: this involves the components of observer variability, both within and between tests, subject variability, and test variability.
5. Sensitive: this is the ability of a test to give a positive finding when the individual screened has the disease or abnormality under investigation.
6. Specific: this is the ability of the test to give a negative finding when the individual does not have the disease or abnormality under investigation.

Rose[7] added the concept of 'yield' which was defined as the number of *new* previously unsuspected cases detected per 100 cases screened. Haggard pointed out that the yield of a screening test declines as case-finding by other means becomes increasingly effective (Fig. 5.1) and coined the term 'incremental yield'.[8]

Formal and opportunistic screening

Formal screening programmes aimed at the whole population are one of the means by which early detection is accomplished, but are not the only method nor necessarily the most important.[9] Opportunistic screening is similar to formal screening, except that the initial contact is initiated by the parents for some other purpose and the professional uses the contact to carry out one or more screening tests or procedures. In contrast with formal screening programmes, opportunistic screening does not incorporate the requirement to seek out all the children in the population so that they can be screened.

Recent changes in attitudes to screening

Research on screening programmes has expanded rapidly in the last few years. There are several reasons for this.

Potential harm

It has been recognized that some screening activities are not merely useless but are potentially harmful because of the unnecessary worry, referrals, and procedures which may result.[10] Indeed, it is unethical to offer screening tests which cannot stand up to critical examination:

In traditional medical practice the patient asks the physician for advice and treatment for his complaint. It is the duty of the physician to do only that for which the patient has given informed consent and to provide care conforming to the standards set by a reasonable body of medical opinion. The patient usually understands, and is often reminded, that diagnostic procedures and treatment may have adverse effects. In screening for asymptomatic or occult disease, on the other hand, the contact is initiated by health care providers, who seek out persons who believe themselves to be well with an offer to optimize their future health. By offering to screen, the physician assumes the same duty of care as would be the case if the patient initiated the contact.[11]

Anxiety

Screening tests and procedures cause anxiety and change people's perceptions about health and normality. People cannot be expected to understand the concept of screening, and are seldom told the implications of a positive test before it is carried out. Parents whose babies have had false-positive screening tests show increased anxiety levels which may persist for weeks or even months after the definitive test shows the baby to be normal. Yet they may feel obliged to participate in the screening programme, sometimes against their own better judgement, because of concerns about potential regrets if a problem should be 'missed'. The phenomenon has been called 'anticipated decision regret'.

Litigation

The increasing readiness of patients to resort to litigation when problems are 'missed' by screening highlights the legal hazards of offering screening tests which are not sufficiently robust to perform the tasks expected of them. Although all professionals resist the idea that their activities should be governed by the fear of litigation, this is an issue that can no longer be ignored. There are already a number of cases in which legal proceedings have been brought because a condition was missed at a screening test. Examples include dislocation of the hip, hypothyroidism, spina bifida occulta, and congenital hearing loss. To offer a screening test or procedure which is insufficiently reliable to

Fig. 5.1 The concept of incremental yield. The diagram refers to detection of hearing loss but could be adapted to any screening programme. It shows the cumulative detection of cases over time. There will usually be a steady trickle of cases detected independent of any screening programme and this is represented by a gradually rising curve during the intervals between screening tests. The incremental yield is the number of new (i.e. previously unrecognized) cases detected *at each successive stage* of the identification programme. In this example, ten cases of congenital hearing loss per 10 000 live births are assumed:

(a) It is assumed that 50 per cent of all cases are found by a neonatal screening test, that 50 per cent of the remainder are found by a screening test at age 7–8 months, and that parents identify a few cases without professional input at random times. The number of cases which remain to be detected after the neonatal screen decreases steadily. The benefits of a screen after 1 year of age (e.g. at 2½) are inevitably small.

(b) It is assumed that there is no neonatal screen and a test at 7–8 months which performs poorly. In this situation, a test at age 2½ has a higher yield.
(Redrawn from Haggard, M. (1993) *Research in the development of effective services for hearing impaired people.* Nuffield Provincial Hospitals Trust, London, by permission of the author and Nuffield Hospitals Trust.)

---

detect the target disorder is not only unethical (see above) but also hazardous from the legal point of view.

The need for information

More information must be provided about existing screening programmes, and any new screening technique must be evaluated not only on the basis of its performance but also from the ethical viewpoint. It should be considered unethical to offer any screening procedure whose validity and potential for causing distress have not been assessed. Parents must have full information and the opportunity to 'opt out' of tests whose purpose they do not understand or accept.

Method of evaluation of screening tests

We examined the screening tests and procedures commonly used in child health surveillance. We attempted to evaluate each test as if it were being proposed now as a new innovation. In some respects, it is more difficult to assess a test which has been in routine use for a long time, but this is not a reason for omitting the exercise. A particular problem was the well-recognized fact that many of the activities examined do not meet the strict criteria for screening tests laid down by

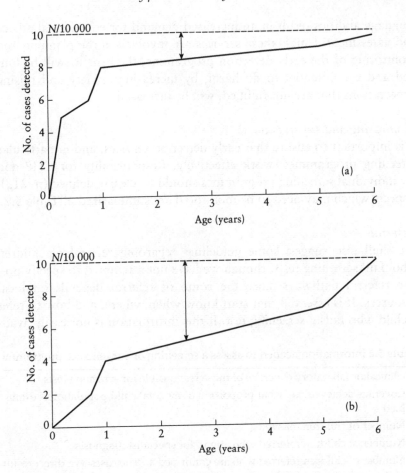

Wilson and Jungner, yet cogent arguments are often adduced for their continued usefulness in the evaluation and care of apparently healthy children.

General principles for the management of screening programmes

Planning and purchasing
Early detection programmes cannot work in isolation. The implications for other aspects of the child's care must always be considered. For instance, screening for hearing loss has major implications for the ear, nose, and throat service, growth monitoring generates additional referrals for paediatric endocrine clinics, and reviews of developmental and

language abilities result in an increased demand for educational advice and assessment. Unless these services are involved in the planning and monitoring of the early detection programme, the benefits will be limited and the potential to do harm, by increasing anxiety and raising expectations that are not fulfilled, will be increased.

Monitoring and supervision
It is important to ensure that early detection services, and in particular screening programmes, work effectively. Responsibility for CHP and for individual screening programmes should be clearly defined (p. 213). Aspects which may need to be monitored are summarized in Table 5.2.

Referral
We shall also suggest some guidelines regarding referral of children who 'fail' screening tests, though we have not attempted to specify precise referral pathways since the route of referral depends on local resources. It is essential that staff know when, where, and how to refer a child who fails a screening test. If this information is not easily avail-

Table 5.2 Information needed to assess a screening or surveillance programme

- Clinical or laboratory expertise of those responsible for screening tests
- Coverage achieved, i.e. what proportion of the total child population is examined
- Number of children referred
- Number of children referred who attend for specialist diagnosis
- Number of children referred who are confirmed as true cases as a direct result of the screening test (yield)
- Number of false positives
- Number of true cases missed
- Number of true cases completing a course of treatment or other intervention
- Number of cases effectively treated
- The impact of the screening programme on other related services
- The delays occurring between each step of the programme and the extent to which these cause or exacerbate parental anxiety
- The quality, accuracy, and readability of the information provided for parents to explain the aims of the programme
- The extent of the benefit accruing to those effectively treated
- The cost of the programme, the cost per case detected, and the value of the benefits obtained
- The training required to initiate the programme and maintain high standards

able, there is a danger that the child may be subjected to repeated tests which fail to produce a definitive diagnosis, or else is lost to follow-up and never receives appropriate treatment.

Notes and references

A more extensive bibliography is available on screening; see p. xi for details.

1. Department of Education and Science (1978). *Warnock report on special educational needs*. HMSO, London.
2. See *Code of Practice*, 1994 (Section 176). HMSO, London. Also consult the two reports of the Audit Commission about pupils with special educational needs: *Getting in on the Act* and *Getting the Act together*. HMSO, London. These are essential reading.
3. Department of Health and Social Security (1972). *Report of a working group on risk registers*. HMSO, London.
4. Holland, W.W. and Stewart, S. (1990). *Screening in health care*. Nuffield Provincial Hospital Trust, London.
5. Wilson, J.M.G. and Jungner, G. (1968). *Principles and practice of screening for disease*. Public Health Papers No. 34, World Health Organization, Geneva.
6. Cochrane, A. and Holland, W. (1969). Validation of screening procedures. *British Medical Bulletin*, 27, 3–8.
7. Rose, G. (1978). *Epidemiology for the uninitiated: screening. British Medical Journal*, 2, 1417–18.
8. Haggard, M. (1993). *Research in the development of effective services for hearing impaired people*, pp. 43–80. Nuffield Provincial Hospitals Trust, London.
9. Hall, D.M.B. and Michel, J.-M. (1995). Screening in infancy. *Archives of Disease in Childhood* 72, 93–6.
10. There is an extensive literature on the psychological problems of screening, e.g. Marteau, T.M. (1990). Screening in practice: reducing the psychological costs. *British Medical Journal* 301, 26–28.
11. Edwards, P. and Hall, D.M.B. (1992). Screening, ethics and the law. *British Medical Journal* 305, 267–8.

6

Physical examination

This chapter covers:

- The neonatal and 6–8 week examinations
- The school entrant examination
- Congenital dislocation of the hip (developmental dysplasia)
- Heart disease
- Hypertension
- Asthma
- Undescended testes and other genital abnormalities

Neonatal and 8-week examinations

The neonate

A thorough physical examination of every neonate is now universally accepted as good practice,[1] and the whole examination can be regarded as a screening procedure with a number of individual components. The yield of this examination is high. It is accepted and expected by parents, and there seems little doubt that they value the reassurance of normality at this time.

The precise timing of the examination is not critical. Local policy should specify how this is to be accomplished in cases where the mother and baby are discharged from hospital within a few hours of birth or the delivery is the sole responsibility of a midwife. In our view a midwife could undertake the neonatal examination, provided that clear guidelines, adequate training, and paediatric support are provided.[2]

For many years a second examination within the first week of life was an accepted routine, but the value of this has been questioned. The yield of significant findings is small, with the possible exception of hip disorders (see below). It seems doubtful whether a formal physical examination at this time would reveal many problems which could not be identified either by the parents or by the midwife and health visitor.

Two months

An examination at around 2 months of age is generally thought to be useful, with a smaller but significant yield of abnormalities. This examination can be done at 8 weeks, to coincide with the revised immunisation schedule though some GPs prefer to do the examination separately, at about six weeks.

The neonatal and 6–8 week examinations are widely believed to be worthwhile, although there is certainly room for considering the precise content and the nature of the procedures used. No other routine physical examinations are so universally accepted, and therefore we decided that physical examinations for screening purposes beyond the age of 8 weeks would require individual justification.

School entrant medical examination

The Working Party was primarily concerned with health surveillance of the preschool population. A detailed review of the literature on the school entrant examination and on school health in general has recently been completed.[3] The yield of significant new physical abnormalities at this examination is generally small. This may in part be attributed to the existence of frequent preschool physical examinations, which should ensure that most significant defects have been discovered by the time that the child goes to school. However, some have argued that the school entrant examination makes an important contribution to child health even if preschool surveillance is working well.

The trend towards a more selective approach to the school medical examination is generally, though not universally, welcomed. A school nurse can undertake a review of previous health care and identify any deficiencies as well as providing health education. She also carries out or coordinates hearing, vision, and height checks.

Nevertheless, it is difficult to achieve high coverage in the immediate preschool period, and a case has been made for universal physical examination of school entrants in areas of high social deprivation and population mobility, or with a large influx of people (e.g. refugees) who have received little or no medical care before entering school. In the latter groups, screening for tuberculosis should also be considered in individuals whose country of origin has a high prevalence of this disease, but screening for other infections and infestations is probably not justified.

It seems obvious that universal school entrant examination would confer *some* benefits. It has been argued that the examination is cheap in terms of cost per child examined, but the cost of identifying one child with a significant new treatable condition is probably high.

Some health authorities also include a developmental examination in their school entrant procedure (Chapter 12).

Individual physical examination procedures

In the following sections we consider individual physical examination procedures which may be used for screening purposes.

Congenital dislocation of the hip

Definition
The term congenital dislocation of the hip (CDH) encompasses a spectrum of conditions in which the head of the femur is, or may be, partly or completely displaced from the acetabulum. It includes dislocation, subluxation, and instability; in addition it may subsume dysplasia of the acetabulum. The term 'developmental dysplasia of the hip' is often preferred to CDH, as it covers a broader range of related conditions and recognizes the importance of the relationships between dysplasia of varying degrees and the stability of the joint.

Causes
The cause of CDH is not known, but genetic factors are important. It is more common in girls. The following factors are associated with an increased risk of CDH: family history in a close relative, breech presentation, postural deformities of the feet, oligohydramnios, and tight swaddling. The first three of these are generally used in identifying a high-risk group for screening purposes (see below).

Incidence
Before neonatal screening was introduced the incidence in Northern European populations of CDH requiring surgery was 0.8–1.6 per 1000, with a mean from a number of studies of around 1.25 per 1000. When the Ortolani–Barlow screening tests for CDH were introduced,

the incidence of neonatal hip instability was reported to be between 2.5 and 20 per 1000, i.e. up to 16 times higher.

Importance of early detection

Some hips are irreducible at birth and will come to surgery however promptly the diagnosis is made, but in most cases the joint is unstable but reducible. Early detection of these is thought to be worthwhile because conservative treatment, commencing within the first 6–8 weeks of life, is often successful, produces better results, and may avoid the need for surgery. Some infants will respond to conservative treatment if started at any time in the first 6 months, but the probability of success decreases with age and the risk of avascular necrosis rises. Thus there is a degree of urgency about the diagnosis and prompt referral of suspect cases is mandatory.

Universal screening for CDH

This was first recommended in 1969, but subsequent research raised doubts about its effectiveness and the topic was reviewed in detail in 1986. Much new work has been published since then, but there is still controversy over the role and effectiveness of screening.[4] The aim of a screening programme for CDH is to ensure normal development and function of the hip by the end of the adolescent growth period.[5]

Management of hip instability

Splintage is usually recommended for hip instability in the belief that this will avoid the need for surgery later on. However, since the rate of neonatal hip instability is up to 16 times higher than that for CDH in unscreened populations, it is obvious that many babies must be splinted unnecessarily. This has disadvantages in cost, both to the health service and to the family, and in the risk of complications such as avascular necrosis of the femoral head and pressure sores.

In some centres, the introduction of neonatal screening is said to have resulted in a substantial fall in the number of babies needing surgery, but in others the rate remains unchanged. The reasons for the discrepancy probably include differences in the age(s) at which screening is performed and the skill and training of those performing the examination. Some research reports suffer from incomplete case ascertainment; it is difficult to ensure that all late cases have been identified, since no single data source provides a complete list of all children requiring treatment for CDH.

The screening tests

Clinical examination detects dislocation, subluxation, and instability; ultrasound can also detect dysplasia. Evaluation of CDH screening is complicated by the lack of a definitive diagnostic test and uncertainty about the natural history.

1. The simplest method of screening is the use of a *checklist of risk factors*. Breech presentation, family history in any relative, and foot deformity are thought to be the most useful. However, a screening policy based only on these high-risk factors will miss many cases.

2. Clinical examination of every baby using the *Ortolani–Barlow manoeuvre* can be performed up to the age of 6–8 weeks. Any baby with a hip which is subluxable or dislocated must be referred, but there is no agreement as to whether 'clicking' hips are significant. Nor is there any clear evidence as to when this examination should be performed or how many times it should be repeated. Instability identified at the neonatal clinical examination may be clinically undetectable at 2 weeks, but ultrasound may reveal that the hip is still dislocated. Conversely, an ultrasound examination later in the first week may reveal dislocation in a significant number of babies who have been passed by an expert examiner as clinically normal in the first 24 hours.

3. *Limited abduction and asymmetric skin creases* are found in many babies with CDH and are sometimes identified first by the parent. These signs should be sought whenever the hips are examined, although they are rarely detected in the neonatal period and are more important after 6–8 weeks of age. The literature lacks any operational definition of 'limited abduction' or any appraisal of the probable referral rates if this physical sign were to be more actively sought. Some babies have asymmetry for other reasons, and abduction may be difficult to assess in active or restless babies. These signs are less obvious in babies with bilateral CDH. Because of these limitations, together with the uncertainties about early treatment mentioned previously, assessment of these signs does not fulfil strict criteria for a screening test. Nevertheless, they are the main means of detecting late or missed cases and make a significant contribution to case finding. It would be undesirable and unwise at present to abandon any further checks after

the first 2 months of life. The options are (a) to seek these signs at the time of the second or third immunization or (b) to do so at the review carried out at 6–9 months. Option (b) is the current practice, although we are aware of one local audit suggesting that option (a) might be a practical alternative and this would have the advantage of earlier detection.

4. The *gait* should be observed once the child is walking, and any child thought to have a limp or the gait abnormality associated with bilateral CDH must be referred.

5. Appraisal of *screening by ultrasound scanning* of the hip is complicated by the existence of two methods, the Graf static approach and the Clarke–Harcke dynamic method. Ultrasound scanning of the hip has been used as (a) a primary screen for all babies or (b) a selective primary screen for babies with risk factors; options (a) and (b) are designed to make sure that cases are not missed. In option (c) it is used as a secondary screen to decide which babies with physical signs need splintage, i.e. to reduce 'overtreatment'. Option (a), if performed in the neonate before discharge, would result in considerable overdiagnosis of unstable hips which would resolve spontaneously, whereas if deferred until 2 weeks it would present considerable logistic problems and incur high costs, which cannot currently be justified as there is no clear evidence of benefit. A popular option at present is a combination of (b) and (c). However, even in the most expert hands, some babies are probably splinted unnecessarily, some cases are still missed, and some who are splinted still require surgery. It is not yet certain that those cases considered *not* to need treatment as a result of the ultrasound findings will invariably have a good outcome, and this is the subject of a current research programme.

Screening policy
The 1986 Expert Working Party pointed out that 'it is impossible to detect every CDH at birth . . . and there must be continuing surveillance until the child is seen to be walking normally'. They recommended that (a) all infants should have an examination for CDH within 24 hours of birth, at the time of discharge from the hospital or within 10 days of birth, at 6 weeks of age, at 6–9 months, and at 15–21 months, and (b) the gait should be reviewed at 24–30 months and again at preschool or school entry examination. The time is not yet

right for radical alterations in these recommendations, but we believe that some changes are needed.

Neonatal examination   Although doubts continue to be expressed about the value of neonatal screening, we do not think that this programme could be discontinued except in the context of a randomized trial. (This might be considered in districts where the rate of late diagnosed CDH appears unchanged by comparison with the prescreening era.) For routine practice, risk factors must be reviewed and at least one examination must be performed. Although it is debatable whether the first day is the best time for this, examination of the hips is easily incorporated into the neonatal examination, whereas it is more difficult to ensure that this is done subsequently.

Practical aspects   It is clear from our review that training is vital if CDH screening is to be effective. However, the more people who carry out these procedures, the more difficult it is to ensure a high standard of training and monitoring. The 'Baby Hippy' model is useful for teaching, although it is expensive and easily damaged.

Children with neurological disease   Acquired hip disorders are common in children with movement disorders such as cerebral palsy, but these should be identified by regular monitoring in a specialist clinic and not by neonatal screening.

Heart disease

The birth prevalence of congenital heart disease (CHD) in the UK is said to be 8 per 1000. The birth prevalence of CHD diagnosed in infancy is 6.5 per 1000 live births. Acquired heart disease in childhood is uncommon. The main causes are Kawasaki disease and myocarditis. Rheumatic heart disease is very rare in the Western world.

Early detection
Early detection of CHD is desirable for four reasons.

1. Deterioration may be rapid and catastrophic, and the outcome may be better if the infant is investigated before this occurs.
2. If the diagnosis is missed in the first few weeks of life because the

infant is asymptomatic, the defect may not present until irreversible changes have occurred, for example pulmonary hypertension in children with left to right shunt.

3. Even defects that are trivial in haemodynamic terms may predispose to endocarditis if antibiotic prophylaxis is not recommended for dental and other procedures

4. Missed diagnoses of heart disease distress parents, even if the delay does not result in any harm to the baby.

Identification—special situations and high risk groups

A small but significant and increasing number of defects are detected by antenatal ultrasound screening.[6] With routine ultrasound examination, it is possible to detect those conditions which do not have two equal-sized ventricles (single ventricle, hypoplastic left heart, pulmonary valve atresia with intact septum) at 17–18 weeks. However, the value of antenatal identification of CHD in terms of improved prognosis for the child or help for the parents is not certain. The overall impact on the epidemiology of CHD or the pattern of service provision is likely to be limited, at least within the next few years.

Patent ductus arteriosus (PDA) is very common in premature infants. Most close spontaneously or with treatment, but a few persist beyond the neonatal period and may not be detected until later.

Loud murmurs in an asymptomatic infant may be due to a small ventricular septal defect (VSD), which is benign, but may also be due to valvular stenosis which needs prompt referral.

Children with Down's syndrome constitute a special case. Approximately 40 per cent have CHD, not always accompanied by significant murmurs or other obvious physical signs in infancy. In cases where there is a substantial left to right shunt, the progression to irreversible pulmonary hypertension is unusually rapid. A normal ECG does not exclude CHD. Parents must not be wrongly assured that their Down's child has a normal heart.[7]

There is also an increased incidence of CHD in a wide variety of other dysmorphic syndromes and in association with malformations, and all such children should be checked with particular care. Children suspected of having Marfan's syndrome need cardiological review.

Parents who have had CHD themselves or a previous child with CHD have an increased risk of a further affected child. They should be offered genetic counselling and fetal echocardiography, preferably at a specialist centre.

Hypertrophic obstructive cardiomyopathy (HOCM) is transmitted by a dominant gene. Decisions about the management of the offspring of people with this condition should be made by a cardiologist with experience of managing the disorder and of counselling affected individuals and their families. Neonatal screening is unlikely to be helpful. Screening for HOCM in any young person embarking on intensive physical activity (such as athletics training) has been suggested, but it is rare (0.2 per 1000) and screening is unlikely to be cost-effective.[8]

Routine examination of all children for CHD
Routine examination of the neonate may reveal cyanosis, respiratory distress, or tachypnoea. The incidence of functional murmurs in the neonate has not been established. Even in the most expert hands, many serious defects, such as interrupted aortic arch, coarctation, etc., may be undetectable by physical examination in the first few days of life. Professionals and parents need to be aware that *normal findings in the newborn infant do not guarantee that the cardiovascular system is normal and that serious heart conditions can present at any time in the first few weeks of life.*[9]

Infants with serious CHD may present with failure to thrive, tachypnoea (particularly if it interferes with feeding), persistent recession, chest infection, sweating, cyanosis, or any combination of these. (Tachypnoea cannot be defined precisely, but in babies under 6 months of age a respiratory rate persistently above 55 is suspicious[10] and, over the age of 4 weeks, the rate should not exceed 30 when asleep.)

Examination of infants at 6–8 weeks of age
The cardiovascular system (CVS) should be examined during the review carried out at between 6 and 8 weeks of age. It is important that this is thorough, and it must include more than simply auscultation for murmurs. The symptoms and signs of CHD listed in the previous paragraph should be sought with care.

Further examinations
The Working Party considered whether examination of the CVS at any time after the 6–8 week review would be of sufficient value to be regarded as a screening test. Conditions which might remain asymptomatic for many years include atrial septal defect (ASD) and isolated

coarctation of the aorta. The physical signs of small ASDs are subtle and would probably be very difficult for a non-specialist to detect at a routine 'screening' examination.

Most patients with coarctation are either symptomatic early in life or present later with hypertension (see p. 105). The majority have abnormal femoral pulses and many have a murmur medial to the left scapula, but we are not aware of any systematic study of examining the femoral pulses in a community setting and therefore do not think that this can be regarded as a screening test. It is good practice to check the femoral or dorsalis pedis pulses as part of a clinical examination, although they can be difficult to feel in toddlers and may occasionally be palpable even when coarctation is present. In a child with symptoms or signs compatible with cardiac disease absence of the femoral pulses is significant, but otherwise the finding should be recorded and a further check made when convenient. On present evidence, missing coarctation in a primary care setting should not be construed as negligent.[11]

Innocent murmurs
The most common problem in routine auscultation of the heart is the difficulty experienced by non-specialist staff in distinguishing innocent from pathological murmurs. Innocent murmurs are very common, occurring in 50 per cent or more of children. They are more often present and prominent in the febrile child. The diagnosis of an innocent murmur in the neonate is more difficult and usually requires the exclusion of CHD.[12]

The characteristics of innocent murmurs include a low intensity, a musical quality, localization to a small area of the precordium, and, most important, absence of any other symptoms or signs referable to the CVS. In this situation there need not be undue concern about overlooking organic heart disease. Conditions which might present with a soft murmur and no other findings include a small ASD, mild pulmonary stenosis, a prolapsing mitral valve, and a bicuspid aortic valve. These lesions are unlikely to be of haemodynamic significance. The risk of endocarditis is very small, and antibiotic prophylaxis to cover dental extraction would only be advised for bicuspid aortic valves.

Referral
Infants with symptoms and signs of CHD need prompt referral for paediatric assessment. It is more difficult to suggest guidance on the refer-

ral of older infants and children with murmurs of uncertain significance in the absence of other signs. Nevertheless, where there is genuine doubt, expert consultation is preferable to leaving parents in a
state of uncertainty. Referral to a paediatrician is probably the best
option, although the advice of a paediatric cardiologist will still be
required occasionally. Echocardiography is helpful in expert hands, but
in small infants defects may easily be overlooked by non-specialist
staff.

Primary prevention

There is so far very little scope for primary prevention of CHD. With
the decline of rheumatic heart disease in the Western world, the most
common cause of acquired heart disease in children in the UK is now
Kawasaki disease.

Hypertension

Screening for asymptomatic evaluation of blood pressure could be justified on two grounds.

1. It would allow detection of secondary hypertension due, for exam-
    ple, to coarctation of the aorta, endocrine disorders, or silent renal
    disease, at a stage before the child presents with serious symptoms
    such as encephalopathy or vision disturbances. The incidence of
    symptomatic hypertension is less than 0.1 per cent (1 in 1000).
2. A screening programme would also detect children with mild eleva-
    tions of blood pressure who have an increased risk of developing
    essential hypertension in adult life. They could be advised to make
    appropriate changes in diet, weight, and lifestyle (although there is
    as yet no evidence that such advice would be either acceptable or
    effective).

The main argument against screening is that there is no clear distinction between normal and elevated readings, and therefore an arbitrary
cut-off point for referral has to be selected. Many children with mild
elevations of blood pressure must be identified and investigated in
order to detect the few with secondary hypertension. Since the former
group cannot be offered any simple treatment programme of proven
effectiveness, there is at present a substantial risk that the harm done
by producing anxiety may exceed any possible benefits.

In an American study on community screening the examination of 10 000 children did not yield a single case of secondary hypertension and no case with primary or essential hypertension was found in which it was thought justifiable to embark on drug treatment. The authors of the study, and subsequently the USA Task Force on screening, concluded that screening for hypertension in childhood could not be recommended. However, it should be noted that children in the USA are examined more frequently by their personal physician than is the case in the UK, and therefore hypertension might be diagnosed at an earlier stage even without a screening programme.)

A more recent American survey proposed that children whose initial reading is above the 95th centile should be re-examined and considered for treatment; however, four out of five such children will be found to have a blood pressure within the normal range on subsequent readings. The more frequently children are examined, the more likely it is that at least one measurement will be elevated. Two further British reviews have concluded that screening for hypertension is not justified at present.[13]

Asthma

With the increasing awareness of asthma and the apparent rise in incidence over the past few years, it has become clear that the definition of 'mild asthma' is difficult.[14] Concordance between different ways of confirming the diagnosis is less than was previously thought, and longitudinal studies suggest that at the mild end of the spectrum bronchial hyper-reactivity may be a temporary or transient phenomenon.[15] Current evidence does not support the introduction of any formal screening programme for asthma.

Primary prevention[16]

There is a little evidence that rigorous allergen avoidance in infants at high risk of atopy will reduce the incidence of allergic disease, at least in the short term. Smoking by the mother in pregnancy increases the risk that the infant will develop asthma and demonstrate increased bronchial hyper-reactivity on histamine challenge. There is controversy as to whether exposure to cigarette smoke (passive smoking) actually causes asthma. It is associated with a reduction in the size of the lungs and smaller airways, and an increased rate of hospital admission for respiratory illness. Reduction in air pollution may also be an important primary preventive measure.

Abnormalities of the genitalia

Careful inspection of the genitalia to detect undescended testicle, hypospadias, ambiguous genitalia and other anomalies is an essential part of the routine neonatal examination. Concerns about medical indications for circumcision (which are often unfounded), and the diagnosis of hernia and hydrocoele, are other common problems raised either by the parents or at a routine examination.

By far the most common problem detectable by screening examination is abnormal descent of the testicle.[17] At birth, 6.0 per cent (60 per 1000) of males have one or both testes undescended, and the rate is some five times higher in low birth-weight babies compared with full-term infants.

A high proportion of testes undescended at birth have descended normally by 3 months of age. The prevalence at this age is 1.6 per cent (16 per 1000). Further natural descent is unlikely after this age. Some testes, although apparently normally descended at 3 months, may be found to be incompletely descended when re-examined between 1 and 5 years of age. The majority of these boys have had late initial descent of the testes between birth and 3 months of age, or have been judged to have incomplete initial descent at the first examination.

Infant boys thought to have incomplete descent of the testis should be referred for surgical opinion before the age of 18 months because early surgery may improve fertility. Orchidopexy probably does not reduce the risk of malignancy associated with the condition, though it may facilitate early diagnosis.

The screening test is a physical examination. The testis is gently manipulated into the lowest position along the pathway of normal anatomical descent without tension being applied. The most precise criterion for diagnosis of undescended testis at birth and in the first few months of life is that the centre of at least one testis should be less than 4 cm below the pubic tubercle, or 2.5 cm in babies weighing under 2.5 kg. Subjective classification by experienced examiners into three categories (well down, high scrotal, or suprascrotal) is as reliable as actual measurement.

Recommendations

Routine reviews

- We recommend the continuation of the **neonatal physical examinations for every baby.**
- We recommend that, with respect to the **school entrant medical examination**, the advice set out in the Report on the Health Care Needs of School Age Children should be followed[3].
- The **6–8 week review** should be continued (see Chapter 14, p. 227) for further discussion of how this should be done).

Congenital dislocation of the hip (developmental dysplasia)

- One individual should be identified to act as **coordinator** for training and quality monitoring.
- The **pathway of referral** and the responsibility for investigation and management of suspected hip disorders in infants, and of infants with risk factors for CDH, should be agreed by specialists and primary care staff, clearly defined, and streamlined to ensure that delays do not occur. This is particularly important at the 6–8 week review, since there may be some urgency in commencing treatment for a newly discovered case at this age.
- The **district coordinator** (p. 214) should ensure that each neonate is assessed for risk factors, and examined once, preferably within the first 48 hours and certainly within the first week, by someone who has been trained to recognize abnormalities.
- Every baby should have a further review of risk factors and an examination of the hips at **6–8 weeks** (p. 227).
- A child with a suspect clinical examination should not be subjected to repeated checks or reviews but **referred promptly.**
- The **list of risk factors** must include family history, breech presentation, and foot deformity. Missed CDH in an infant with a positive family history is particularly distressing for parents and may result in litigation.
- When the coordinator is confident that these two examinations are competently performed, the additional benefits and practicality of carrying out a **second examination within the first 2 weeks** should be assessed. If this is undertaken, the results should be monitored.

Options for performing this examination might include the midwife (at the same time as the Guthrie test), the health visitor (at her first visit), or the general practitioner.

- **Parents should be warned** (for example in the personal child health record) that no screening procedure is perfect, and informed about the physical signs of hip disorders, i.e. limited abduction, asymmetry and limp. They should be told whom to contact if they have any concerns.
- **Limited abduction and asymmetry** should be actively sought at least once after the 6–8 week review; this is most conveniently done between 6 and 9 months of age but could be carried out at the same time as the third immunization.
- The observation of any **gait abnormalities** suggestive of CDH at the 18–24 month review should lead to referral.
- **Secondary ultrasound screening** is in widespread use at present. Scanning babies with clinically unstable hips, or risk factors, at or after 2 weeks of age is the option preferred in most districts. Nevertheless, the evidence is not yet conclusive. Districts proposing to introduce this technique should, if possible, do so in the context of a controlled trial.
- **Universal screening by ultrasound** cannot be recommended except in the context of a research programme.

Monitoring the screening programme

The priority at present is the setting and monitoring of quality standards for examination, recording, referral, and treatment. The training of staff is a priority, and the 'Baby Hippy' model (which has recently been reintroduced by the manufacturers) enables staff to learn the correct technique.

Process measures include the coverage of screening, numbers referred for specialist opinion at each age, and numbers of babies needing treatment with splints or surgery. Quality measures should also include the intervals between referral and specialist consultation, and between consultation and treatment (when needed). The presumed benefit and therefore the best outcome measure for CDH screening is reduction in hip morbidity in adult life, but radiographic appearances of the joint at age two may be an acceptable proxy measure. Monitoring of late diagnosed cases is useful as a warning of deficiencies in the system, but numbers in any one district are too small to permit generalizable conclusions.

Further research

A number of authorities continue to express disquiet about screening for CDH, and it is clear that more research is required. A trial is currently being undertaken by the Medical Research Council to assess the benefits and hazards of ultrasound screening. Although randomized trials are expensive and present considerable difficulties, they may be the only way to answer the questions raised above.

Heart disease

- Symptoms and signs of CHD should be routinely sought at **the newborn examination** and at **the review at 6–8 weeks of age**.

- Parents should be aware of the significance of potentially serious symptoms, notably **persistent tachypnoea**, and should be encouraged to seek help if concerned. This information could be provided through the personal child health record.

- All professionals dealing with children should be familiar with the symptoms and signs of cardiac disease in babies, and in particular with the risk of **rapid deterioration** in infancy once the child presents with symptoms.

- After the 6–8 week review, the CVS should be examined in any child with **relevant complaints** and on **an opportunistic basis** when the child is examined for other reasons.

- The potential benefits of routine examination of the CVS after 8 weeks of age do **not** justify any more specific recommendation.

- Children with conditions having a high risk of CHD, notably **Down's syndrome**, should have an ECG and an echocardiogram in the first few weeks of life.

- Primary health care teams should be reminded about the importance of early diagnosis and referral of **Kawasaki disease**.

- There is **no** justification for carrying out a **'screening' check for heart murmurs** after 8 weeks of age.

Hypertension

We recommend that at present **no** attempt should be made to introduce universal screening for hypertension. Further research on the detection of secondary hypertension and the prevention of essential hypertension may eventually change this view. Measurement of blood pressure must be part of the clinical evaluation of any child presenting with a relevant medical problem.

Asthma

- **Primary prevention** by reducing parental smoking should be pursued and is one of the many reasons for addressing this issue in health promotion programmes.
- In view of the variability in symptoms of mild asthma, and the lack of sensitivity, specificity, and reproducibility of tests for bronchial hyper-reactivity, we do **not** think that a screening programme could fulfil the Wilson and Jungner criteria (p. 83).

Undescended testes

- A note should be made of **testicular descent** at the neonatal and 8-week examinations. The second examination is particularly important in those cases where the testis is *not* 'well down' in the scrotum.
- **No further check** need be made as a matter of routine. Parents can be shown how to check testicular descent themselves (for example while the child is in the bath).
- If there is doubt about the descent of either or both testes after 6–8 weeks, the child should be **referred for surgical opinion** to a surgeon with experience of and interest in paediatric surgery.
- **Explicit guidelines** are needed to ensure that the system works efficiently. These will depend on local circumstances, but we suggest that the referral should be made immediately after the 6–8 week examination, the surgical clinic appointment should be sent so that the child can be seen before his first birthday, the general practitioner should be notified of non-attenders, and any deliberate delay in sending the parents an appointment should not be incorporated in measures of clinic waiting list times.
- These checks are often neglected in children who are disabled. *All* children should be examined, although judgement is needed as to when treatment is desirable.
- The age of diagnosis and treatment, and the number of boys discovered to have an untreated undescended testis at the age of 5 or

subsequently, can be **recorded as a measure of success** in screening for undescended testes.

• **Training** for primary care staff should include the indications for circumcision and the recognition and management of hernia and hydrocele.

Notes and references

A more extensive bibliography is available on CDH, heart disease, and other topics; see p. xi for details.

1. Moss, G.D., Cartlidge, P.H.T., Speidel, B.D., and Chambers, T.L. (1991). Routine examination in the newborn period. *British Medical Journal* 302, 878–9.
2. Mackeith, N. (1995). Who should examine the normal neonate? *Nursing Times* 91(14), 34–5.
3. Polnay, L. (1995). *The health care needs of school aged children*. British Paediatric Association, London.
4. For a comprehensive review, see Leck, I. (1995). Congenital dislocation of the hip. In *Antenatal and neonatal screening* (ed. N. Wald). Oxford University Press.
5. A useful collection of articles on CDH appears in *Journal of Pediatric Orthopedics*, Part B 2(2) (1994).
6. Cullen, S., Sharland, G.K., Allan, L.D., and Sullivan, I.D. (1992). Potential impact of population screening for prenatal diagnosis of congenital heart disease. *Archives of Disease In Childhood* 67, 775–8.
7. Tubman, T.R., Shields, M.D., Craig, B.G., Mulholland, H.C., and Nevin, N.C. (1991). Congenital heart disease in Down's syndrome: two year prospective early screening study. *British Medical Journal*, 302, 1425–7.
8. A collection of papers on HOCM appears in *British Medical Journal*, 310, 856–60 (1995).
9. Abu-Harb, M., Hey, E., and Wren, C. (1994). Death in infancy from unrecognised congenital heart disease. *Archives of Disease in Childhood* 71, 3–7.
10. Morley, C.J., Thornton, A.J., Fowler, M.A., Cole, T.J., and Hewson, P.H. (1990). Respiratory rate and severity of illness in babies under 6 months old. *Archives of Disease In Childhood* 65, 834–7.
11. Thoele, D.G., Muster, A.J., and Paul, M.H. (1987). Recognition of coarctation of the aorta. A continuing challenge for the primary care physician. *American Journal of Diseases of Children* 141, 1201–4.
12. Jordan, S.C. (1994). Innocent murmurs—when to ask a cardiologist. *Current Paediatrics* 4, 59–61.
13. de Swiet, M. and Dillon, M.J. (1989). Hypertension in children. *British Medical Journal* 299, 469–470.
14. Primhak, R. and Powell, C. (1994). Screening for asthma in schoolchildren. *Paediatric Respiratory Medicine* 2(1), 6–8. (Sets out the arguments against screening for asthma.)

15. Martinez, F.D. (1995). Asthma and wheezing in the first six years of life. *New England Journal of Medicine* 332, 133–8. (A reassuring review of the prognosis for wheezy infants.)
16. Cullinan, P., and Newman Taylor, A.J. (1994). Asthma in children: environmental factors. *British Medical Journal* 308, 1585–6.
17. John Radcliffe Hospital Cryptorchidism Study Group, (1988). Clinical diagnosis of crytorchidism. *Archives of Disease in Childhood* 63, 587–91.
    Eardley, I. Saw, K.C. and Whitaker, R.H. (1994). Trapped and ascending testes. *British Journal of Urology* 73, 204–6.

7
Growth monitoring

This chapter:
- Reviews the value of growth monitoring
- Outlines the reasons why growth monitoring may be useful
- Describes the requirements for successful growth monitoring
- Makes recommendations for growth monitoring
- Examines the value of measuring the head circumference

Value of growth monitoring

Screening or monitoring?

With the possible exception of single height measurements (p. 119), weighing and measuring children cannot be regarded as screening and therefore we have adopted the term 'growth monitoring' (GM).

Is growth monitoring useful?

Although the routine measurement of height, weight, and head circumference is widely accepted, and strongly supported by most health professionals, there is still disagreement about the ages when measurements are made or recorded and the threshold at which referral for specialist advice is desirable. Interpretation of the measurements requires skill and judgment, and is easier when several measurements are taken over a period of time. It is important not to overlook children with growth disorders, but inappropriate referrals generate both parental anxiety and a substantial increase in specialist workload.

Recent experience in developing countries[1] suggests that, although universally encouraged as a health promotion measure, GM does not necessarily have a significant impact on the health of children. GM in developing nations relies mainly on weight rather than height measurement and is mainly directed at the problem of malnutrition; nevertheless, the reasons for the lack of impact are probably relevant in the industrialized nations as well as in the developing world. They include incomplete coverage (the families whose children might benefit most from GM are those with multiple social and economic problems, who have difficulty in making full use of preventive health care measures), inaccurate weighing, charting, and interpretation, rushed or inaccurate counselling of parents owing to inadequate staff training, poverty (lack of money and/or social support enabling parents to implement the advice given), and cultural resistance to particular dietary recommendations.

Benefits of growth monitoring

The potential advantages of GM can be listed as follows:

- *Detecting disorders* GM may facilitate the early detection of a variety of disorders (see box).
- *Health promotion* GM is a tool which can be used to assess and inform health promotion activity in respect of nutritional advice and overall quality of child care. For example, impaired growth may be associated with child neglect or abuse.
- *A focus of interest for parents* GM is valued by parents and is used by them as a focus for visits to the clinic or surgery. Regular GM may be useful to reassure the parents that the child is thriving. The baby's weight gain is often used as a discussion point regarding nutrition and other aspects of child rearing. Similarly, parents take some satisfaction from recording their child's growth in height.
- *Public health aspects* Information about child growth in the whole population may be useful in several ways. First, there is a tendency for children to be taller in successive generations (the so-called 'secular trend'), though this is now levelling off. Second, in the last few years data collected half a century ago have been used to establish links between growth in fetal life and early infancy, and disease patterns in the adult.[2] Third, since there is a link between height and social circumstances, GM provides a window on the effects of poverty and changing social inequalities.

The relationships between the size of children at any given age, their genetic background, and their social circumstances are complex. Growth patterns may to some extent reflect not only the circumstances of the present generation but also the social deprivation experienced in childhood by their parents and even their grandparents. Thus contemporary population growth data is of limited value in assessing the *current* public health of the population.

Conditions detectable by growth monitoring

Hypothyroidism (juvenile)—incidence uncertain. Most congenital hypothyroidism is detected by neonatal screening but a few cases are inevitably missed. Juvenile hypothyroidism is more common in girls and is usually autoimmune in nature.

Growth hormone insufficiency (GHI)—incidence 1 in 3000–5000. GHI can occur in association with other disorders, but isolated or idiopathic GHI is the most common. It can present in early infancy as a short baby, sometimes accompanied by microphallus and/or hypoglycaemia, or as short stature in early or mid-childhood. Late-onset GHI can be difficult to differentiate from the physiological deficiency of growth hormone which may occur with delayed puberty. Because of this variable age of presentation, no single screening test could be expected to identify every case of GHI.

Turner's syndrome—incidence at least 1 in 2500 females. Less than 50 per cent of cases are identified at birth, but in the remainder short stature or primary amenorrhoea are the presenting features. If tall parents have a child with Turner's syndrome, she may not necessarily be identified as short, i.e. below the 0.4 centile, by a single measurement, but the growth chart will show that the height is crossing centiles.

Growth impairment can be the presenting feature of many other disorders. The majority are likely to be associated with other symptoms, but short stature may be the only sign of conditions such as coeliac disease, inflammatory bowel disease, or chronic renal failure.

Cranial or total body irradiation and intracranial tumours These children should be under specialist care but occasionally they are 'missed' or lost to follow up.

Syndromes such as Russell–Silver syndrome or Noonan's syndrome may be identified as a result of growth impairment or short (or tall) stature.

Some forms of bone dysplasia can present with short stature, but without other obvious disproportion in the early stages. Diagnosis is important because genetic counselling may be required and new possibilities for treatment are being investigated.

Short normal children ('idiopathic short stature') should currently only be treated with growth hormone in the context of clinical trials. Short-term improvement in height has been shown clearly, but the long-term benefits and hazards are still unknown.

Growth monitoring might also be useful as a means of detecting excessively *tall stature*.

Such data clearly are important but to be useful they must be reliable, carefully documented and preserved for the future. Secure long-term funding for a small number of GM projects in districts with a declared interest and track record in this field would seem to be a more logical investment than monitoring growth in every district.

Weight monitoring

'Normal' weight gain is reassuring to parents. Satisfactory weight gain does not rule out growth disorders; for example, growth hormone deficiency and hypothyroidism may be associated with normal or even increased weight gain.

Slow weight gain

Relative undernutrition may occur in many situations such as weaning difficulties, late weaning, minor illness, and family disturbances, and this may be associated with short periods of slow weight gain or temporary weight loss. Prolonged failure to gain weight or continuing weight loss are more likely to have serious implications. However, it is rare that the weight chart is the only clue to a serious abnormality affecting growth in infancy. Other symptoms or signs are nearly always present as well, and in their absence hospital admission is rarely helpful since the investigation of infants whose only problem is slow weight gain seldom reveals any significant organic disease.

Babies whose line of weight gain crosses centile channels downwards are often diagnosed as 'failing to thrive' (FTT). This term should only be used when there is evidence that the slow weight gain is abnormal *for that baby*. There is no simple way of assessing whether a particular growth pattern is outside the limits of 'normality', although the height and build of the parents should of course be taken into account when assessing a clinical problem.[3]

Most babies who gain weight slowly or whose weight graph gradually crosses centile lines downwards are simply adopting their own genetically determined growth trajectory. There is no reason to assume that every baby should continue on the same centile from birth onwards. Similarly, there is wide variation in the relationship between weight and length.

About 50 per cent of babies cross at least one channel on the weight chart between 6 weeks of age and 12 or 18 months. Up to 5 per cent fall across two channels. Babies who are large at birth are more likely to show falls of this magnitude. On average, small babies catch up and large babies catch down. This is explained by the phenomenon of 'regression to the mean' (see Appendix A). Deprivation and poverty increase the risk that a child will grow at a rate below genetic potential, but substantial centile shifts are seen in babies of all social classes.

There is concern that babies with poor weight gain may have subtle feeding difficulties which might benefit from expert intervention, and also that they might be at increased risk of neglect, abuse, long-term developmental problems, and cardiovascular disease in adult life. Poor weight gain might also herald sudden infant death, though this relationship has proved to be insufficiently robust to be of practical value.

Failure to thrive

The identification of FTT is often regarded as the main justification for continued weight monitoring, mainly because psychosocial factors are sometimes associated with poor growth which in this situation is known as 'non-organic failure to thrive' (NOFTT). In severe cases of suspected NOFTT, hospital admission or placement with a foster parent may result in a dramatic growth spurt, confirming the impression of insufficient food intake and an inadequate environment. However, such cases are the exception. Only a minority of children with very slow weight gain subsequently suffer abuse or neglect.

Deciding whether a baby with slow weight gain should be regarded as failing to thrive can be difficult. Management decisions must be made on the basis of the whole clinical picture rather than from the weight chart alone. Parents must not be subjected to unjustified worry, and unnecessary advice and intervention. Supportive management with community-based nutritional and psychological advice is probably beneficial. Very frequent weighing can be counterproductive as it often reveals fluctuations week by week even though there is an upward trend. This may result in desperate attempts by the parents to increase the baby's food intake, leading in turn to further feeding difficulties.

The 'overweight' baby

Crossing centiles in an upwards direction may also cause concern. This reflects an outdated view that infant obesity might be an important, and preventable, risk factor for adult obesity. It is rarely necessary or useful to comment adversely on the fact that a baby looks chubby or fat.

Interpretation of centile shifts in infancy

A new type of chart ('conditional reference charts') will soon be available. This will enable staff to assess the probability that a given rate of weight gain is abnormal, but the correct use and interpretation of such charts will need a good understanding of infant growth, and further staff training will be essential.

Conclusion

Growth should be monitored by length measurement as well as weight in any baby where there is concern, and in all children as soon as standing height can be measured around the age of 2 years. As a routine procedure, however, there seems little justification for regular weighing once the parent and primary care team are satisfied that the baby is feeding normally and has begun to gain weight. We are not convinced that the advantages conferred by regular weighing after the first few months of life justify the resources required or the anxiety generated by uncertain or inexpert interpretation of growth charts.

Whatever professionals may think, parents will continue asking for facilities for their babies to be weighed or to weigh the baby themselves. When parents or other relatives are anxious about their child's weight or food intake, plotting the child's weight on a chart may be useful as a way of reassuring them.

Length and height monitoring

Length

We are doubtful about the value of routinely measuring length in the neonate, although this is essential if *any* abnormality is suspected. The logistics of ensuring that accurate measurements are made on all babies would become increasingly difficult with the rising number of home deliveries and very short hospital stays.

A 'baseline' length measurement at 6–8 weeks of age could be accomplished with much less difficulty. The main benefit of this would be identification of very short babies (length below the 0.4 centile), for example those with severe endocrine deficiency disorders, skeletal dysplasias, or Silver–Russell syndrome.

It has been suggested that a measurement of length taken at birth or at 6–8 weeks might subsequently be useful in difficult diagnostic situations. However, there is as yet no convincing evidence that records of one or more routine length measurements throughout the first year of life would simplify the differential diagnosis of FTT or growth disorders.

Height

Many children with short stature are identified by parents or by paediatricians caring for the child because of other medical conditions. However, monitoring of height might be justified by the following considerations.

- It is important to monitor growth (weight *and* length/height) in cases where some abnormality is suspected, for example in an infant who at birth was noted to be very small for dates, or who is thought to be failing to thrive, or who has a dysmorphic syndrome. Children who suffered from intrauterine growth retardation may grow more slowly and gain weight at a lower rate than normal. Research is currently being undertaken to assess possible ways of treating these children.

- It might permit the early detection of conditions which limit growth but may not be accompanied by any other symptoms or signs, for example growth hormone insufficiency, hypothyroidism, or Turner's syndrome (see box on p. 111). The early identification of short stature associated with hormonal deficiencies is particularly important because early treatment improves the prognosis for adult height.

- GM might facilitate the detection of conditions causing unusually rapid growth, for example congenital adrenal hyperplasia, thyrotoxicosis, precocious puberty, etc.

- Although we focused primarily on the preschool years, the opportunity was taken to consider which universal screening and monitoring procedures might be useful in the school years. There is increasing interest in the treatment of constitutional delay in growth and puberty (CDGP), but we concluded that professional awareness of the problem and of treatment possibilities is more important at present than a formal monitoring programme.

Requirements for successful growth monitoring

Effective GM depends on all the following factors:[4],[5]

- availability of suitable growth charts (see box);
- correct measurement techniques;
- accurate transfer of measurements to chart;

The Tanner Whitehouse growth charts are now outdated because:

- There has been a trend over the last few decades for children to grow taller (the so-called 'secular trend').
- It has been noted in the last few years that weight gain in early infancy is often more rapid than is indicated on the charts and this is followed by apparent growth faltering. This is probably because of changes in feeding practices, notably a higher incidence of breastfeeding and the use of improved or 'humanized' milk formula.

The nine-centile growth charts first published in 1993 (Fig. 7.1) describe current growth patterns more precisely[6] and have two additional advantages:

- Each channel (the interval between each pair of lines on the chart) now represents 0.67 (two-thirds) of a standard deviation, so that crossing a complete channel now has the same significance whatever the initial height of the child.
- The chart now includes a minus and plus 2.67 SD line, equivalent to the 0.4 and the 99.6 centiles respectively. Only one child in 250 lies above or below these lines, whereas the figure is 1 in 44 for the two standard deviation line. A child below the 0.4 centile has a significant probability of having an organic cause for short stature.

The charts were compiled using data for white children only. Growth charts for ethnic minority groups are not thought to be desirable because:

- There would be considerable practical difficulties in assembling a sufficiently large cohort of children from any one ethnic group to produce a reliable chart.
- Ethnic groups differ in the extent and the rate of the 'secular trend' in height and very frequent revisions would be necessary.
- Ethnic groups are not homogeneous (for example, children whose families come from different parts of India show substantial differences in growth patterns and final height).
- Although Afro-Caribbean children tend to be slightly taller and Asian children slightly smaller than white Caucasian children, these differences are best allowed for by consideration of parental heights rather than by ethnic origin.

- correct interpretation (requiring an understanding of normal and abnormal growth);
- time, expertise and resources to explain the measurements to the parents and to initiate appropriate action when necessary;
- access to specialist advice.

Measurement techniques*

Weight
Weight is easy to measure. Modern scales, if properly maintained and checked, weigh to within 10–20 grams. Weight may fluctuate by several hundred grams, depending on the contents of bowel, bladder, and stomach, as well as minor fluctuations due to intercurrent illness.

Length and height measurements
The first 12–18 months of life In this age group it is usual to measure supine length, using a commercially available measuring device. The equipment used in specialist clinics is expensive, but low-cost devices can produce measurements of acceptable accuracy. Although the error of length measurements is greater than that when measuring standing height, useful information can still be obtained because of the higher growth velocity in early infancy. (NB No evidence has been found to support the suggestion that extension of the hips in the neonate, in order to measure length more accurately, has any relationship with dislocation of the hips.)

As soon as the child can stand Delays in treatment of growth disorders result in loss of final height. Ideally, therefore, height measurement should begin as soon as the child can stand; in practice, this means at around the age of 2. Some 2-year-olds are upset by the procedure, and two adults may be needed to obtain a reliable measurement. The 2-year review is often done at home (p. 230) and suitable equipment may not always be available, but measurements can be taken at the surgery or health centre. Most 3-year-olds can be measured without difficulty.

Devices for measuring height A simple 'screening' chart can be used to detect those children who are very short. It has the serious disadvan-

---

* The measuring equipment and growth charts referred to in this chapter can be obtained from the Child Growth Foundation, 2 Mayfield Avenue, London W4 1PW, UK (tel. 0181 994 7625, fax 0181 995 9075).

Difficulties with growth monitoring: accuracy and reproducibility

Inaccurate measurements can be due to:

- Poor installation of equipment
- Inadequate maintenance
- Relocation of portable instruments in a slightly different position each time they are used
- Loose wobbly head pieces on graduated ruler type instruments

These errors can be avoided by checking the location of the instrument with a 1 m measuring stick.

Poor reproducibility

- A correct and standardized measurement technique is important.
- Repeat measurements made on the same child are rarely the same, even when the same instrument is used by the same observer. This problem is not avoided by using more expensive equipment.
- Ninety per cent of the variability is in the children themselves. There is a small diurnal variation (height is greatest on first rising in the morning and decreases during the day with the most rapid decrease during the first hour). Height changes from one moment to the next and there is no exact or 'correct' height for a child.
- Stretching the child by applying gentle upwards pressure under the jaw does not eliminate this source of variability.

Growth velocity estimations do not increase precision because:

- For an experienced observer measuring children under ideal conditions the SD of a single height measurement (SDshm) is around 0.25 cm. For height velocity, two measurements are needed. A child observed to have grown 4 cm between two measurements 1 year apart might in reality have grown between 3.3 cm (very low velocity) and 4.7 cm which is within the normal range (95 per cent confidence limits).
- Under field conditions these limits would be even wider since multiple observers and different conditions and instruments would be used. Differences between observers on the same occasion can be as great as 1.5 cm.
- The rate of growth (growth velocity) varies with age, sex, and initial height.

The problem of bias

Readings of height and weight are subject to bias if the observer knows previous readings or has a preconceived idea as to whether or not the child is growing 'normally'. Ideally, measurements should be taken without knowledge of the previous figure and without prior reference to the growth chart.

Short-term variability

Growth rates vary with the season of the year, intercurrent illnesses, and other factors. Therefore even the most precise measurements made over a short period of time (6 months or less) are likely to be misleading.

tage that no height measurement for future reference is recorded for those children who 'pass' the screening test. Cheap measuring sticks, often mounted on weighing scales, are inaccurate. Measurement errors can be as much as 1–2 cm. For clinic or school use, good results are obtained with a minimeter or Leicester height measuring device. The latter has the advantage that no metre measuring stick is needed to check its accuracy. Although specialist clinics use more robust and expensive equipment, this does not necessarily increase accuracy.

It is often wrongly assumed that height measurement is easy. Reliability has two components—accuracy and reproducibility or precision. Inaccuracy is remediable, but imperfect reproducibility is unavoidable.

Height velocity   It has been suggested that the use of height velocity charts might overcome these difficulties and facilitate the detection of disordered growth. However, growth data plotted on a growth velocity chart are no more informative than the same data correctly plotted on a height chart (see box).

How many measurements? Interpretation of height charts

Charts which show only the third, fifth, or second centile are of limited value for screening as too many false-positive cases are identified. The new nine-centile charts (Figure 7.1), show the 0.4 and 99.6 centiles and, since only one child in 250 will be shorter or taller than this, there is a high probability that any such child has an organic disorder and that it is not due solely to familial factors. Thus if the new charts are used, any single length or height measurement (whether opportunistic or at child health surveillance reviews) could be regarded as a screening test. Its sensitivity would be low, as many children with impaired growth will nevertheless be above the 0.4 centile, at least during the early years of childhood when treatment has the most to offer.

There are fundamental difficulties with interpreting short-term changes in growth patterns. In order to identify the majority of children with growth disorders, long-term growth data are needed to improve reliability by establishing a trend. However, if GM is to include this more ambitious aim, primary care staff must know how to interpret the findings. There can be no simple rule of thumb since, depending on the age of the child and the height of the child when the first measurement is taken, the height line of a normal child may cross one or even two channels. The probability that a given height centile

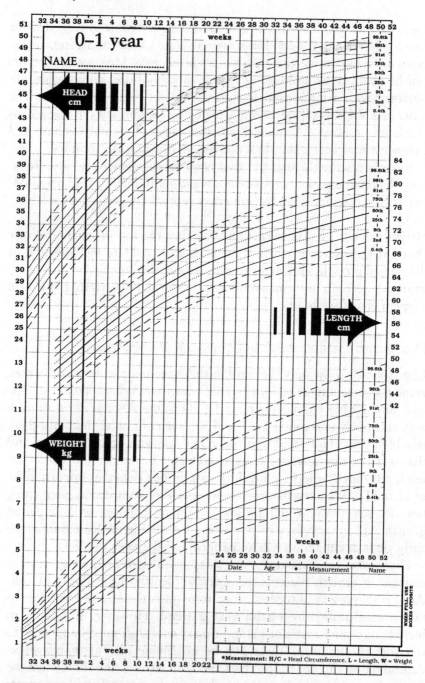

Fig. 7.1 Boys growth chart (0–1 year). © Child Growth Foundation. Available from Harlow Printing, Maxwell Street, South Shields, NE33 4PU, UK.

change over time is normal can be calculated[6]. Whether and how these data could be used to improve the accuracy of referrals is not yet known. The question is particularly important because specialist investigation of short stature is time consuming and can be difficult.

Between half and three-quarters of all children with growth disorders should have been identified by the time that they start school. The number of children remaining to be identified thereafter decreases with each successive age when measurements are taken (incremental yield, p. 86). A further measurement between the ages of 7 and 9 would facilitate detection of conditions in which growth falters in mid-childhood, for example Turner's syndrome, late-onset growth hormone insufficiency, and juvenile-onset hypothyroidism. However, the ratio of true cases discovered to normal short children might be less favourable.

Parental heights
The heights of the parents should be obtained if possible and recorded on the child's growth chart. These measurements may help to decide whether parental size is an adequate explanation for the child's short stature (the procedure is explained on the new growth charts). Parents themselves may have a growth disorder and/or suffered deprivation in their own childhood, and so parental short stature should be interpreted with caution.

Weight and weight for height

Although the main focus of GM after infancy is on height gain and the detection of growth disorders, poor weight gain and obesity may also cause concern to parents and sometimes to professionals. Any child whose health or growth is causing concern should be weighed. Body mass index charts have recently been published[7] and should facilitate the interpretation of weight for height, but further experience will be needed to determine their clinical value.

Recommendations for growth monitoring

- **Staff training** in measurement technique, the interpretation of growth charts (including how to take into account the parental heights), normal growth and its variants, and the management of slow weight gain, FTT, NOFTT, and other disorders is vital.

- There are opportunities to **weigh the baby at each routine visit** for a review or an immunization, and this should be done **if thought necessary** by parent or professional. Accurate weighing requires that the baby be weighed nude unless there are special circumstances (e.g. a dressing or splint). In this case, the state of dress should be recorded. If the baby is weighed naked, the room must be warm.

- The baby may be weighed **at other times if the parent or a professional** considers it necessary.

- Facilities should be provided for the **parents to weigh the baby** when they wish and professional advice should be available to help them interpret the results.

- Primary care staff must have access to **equipment** suitable for length and height measurements and an adequate supply of growth charts.

- Height should be measured with a **Leicester height measure** *or*, if any other device is used, it must be **calibrated** regularly with a 1 metre rule.

- The scales should be checked and **calibrated** regularly.

- All measurements should be entered on the **nine-centile charts**, which should be kept in the personal child health record.

- Correction for **gestational age** is essential up to the age of 2 years.

- Measurements should be **dated**, recorded in figures as well as a point on the graph, and **signed**.

- Any child whose growth is causing **serious concern to his or her parents** should be assessed with care and considered for specialist referral.

- Any child who has a *single* length or height measurement above the 99.6 centile or below the 0.4 centile should be **referred**.

- **In the neonate, length should be measured** if the infant is of low birthweight or if *any* abnormality is suspected.

- **At 6–8 weeks, length should be measured** in any infant who was of low birthweight (less than 2500 grams), if any disorder is suspected or present, and in any infant whose health, growth, or feeding pattern is causing concern. It must be recorded on the chart.

- After 6–8 weeks, further length measurements should be taken when there are **specific indications**.

- A **height measurement should be made** and recorded at around **18–24 months of age**.

- Measurements of height should be made at the further reviews at

around 3.5 years and at or soon after school entry, preferably at about 5 years of age.

- **Two alternative approaches** are suggested for height monitoring after school entry.

  (a) *Selective approach* This would involve a further measurement of height at around 7 to 8 years of age, in the following circumstances: (i) concern about the child's health or growth; (ii) missing or incomplete height data for the preschool years (i.e. less than three measurements between 2 and 5 years); (iii) children whose height at age 5 is on or below the 2SD line (second centile). A decision should then be made as to whether monitoring should be discontinued or should be undertaken in a growth clinic.

  (b) *Universal approach* This would require at least one further height measurement to be recorded on *all* children between 7 and 9 years of age. This approach is strongly supported by endocrine and growth specialists; however, it would require an additional contact in some school health services, and there is little formal evidence of its value. We recommend that it should be undertaken in the context of a well-organized research study (see below) so that the benefits and costs can be assessed.

- Whereas there is no dispute that single measures of height outside the 99.6 or 0.4 centile constitute an indication for referral, the interpretation of channel shifts over time ("slow growers') is more difficult. **Guidelines for this are suggested in Table 7.1** but may need modification in the light of further experience. Height velocity charts do not help to improve the accuracy of growth monitoring and are not recommended.

- Growth monitoring should not be omitted in children with **disabling conditions** and **dysmorphic syndromes**. Growth charts are now available for children with Down's, Turner's, and Noonan's syndromes, and for achondroplasia, and these should be used.

- Meticulous growth data collection and storage for **long-term audit and research** are important and should be supported in those districts where sufficient expertise and commitment exist, but should not currently be regarded as a goal for every district.

- These recommendations may change in the light of further evidence about the treatment of **'normal short' children.**

Table 7.1 Guidelines proposed for identification of slow-growing children

---

1. Pre-school children (less than 5 years, i.e. up to and including school entry:
   - refer if a child's height crosses two channel widths between any pair of measurements;
   - review after a further year if the child's height crosses one or more channel widths, but less than two.
2. School-age children (5–9 years).
   - refer if a child's height crosses one or more channels between any pair of measurements.
   - review after a further year if the height crosses half a channel width or more between any pair of measurements.

We emphasize that these proposals have not been formally tested to determine whether (a) they are useful and acceptable to primary health care team staff and (b) how well they would perform in terms of sensitivity, specificity, and positive predictive value.[8]

Audit

GM should be subject to audit. The quality of measurement and charting, and the action taken when abnormality is suspected, should be reviewed. Crude outcome indicators such as age of starting growth hormone treatment are not helpful because (a) numbers are small in any one district and (b) too many variables affect this indicator. The number of new cases detected by monitoring, their subsequent management, and the reasons for any delay in diagnosis are suitable topics for audit. Growth clinics should monitor their own performance in collaboration with district and tertiary services (see p. 212).

Research

Research is needed on the following topics.

- The definition, identification, and management of slow weight gain, FTT, and NOFTT, and the role and value of conditional reference charts in managing these problems. The relevance of regular weighing to the detection of psychosocial deprivation needs further evaluation.
- A study is needed to determine the yield produced by following the guidelines for height monitoring set out above, in terms of new cases discovered and benefiting from treatment or intervention.

- There are wide variations in existing policy regarding GM in schools. In some districts, annual height measurements are continued to at least the age of 14. This 'natural experiment' could be used to ascertain the benefits of the various policies.
- The optimum approach to service provision needs further study, taking account of the increase in referral rate which will probably accompany more determined efforts to improve early detection.
- Body mass index charts will need evaluation to determine whether and how they contribute to GM and to management decisions.

Head circumference

A routine measurement of head circumference is intended to aid the detection of two groups of disorders, those characterized by a large head and those with a small head. These disorders cannot be diagnosed by measurement of the head circumference alone. Since 2 per cent of children have a head circumference above the 98th centile, and 2 per cent are below the second centile, other evidence must be sought to determine whether a particular measurement is significant.

Conditions with enlargement of the head include hydrocephalus, subdural effusion and haematoma, and a number of less common conditions associated with dysmorphic syndromes, etc.

Hydrocephalus is characterized by a head measurement that is crossing centile lines upwards, together with the well-known features of suture separation, tense fontanelle, prominent veins, downward gaze, irritability, and sometimes developmental abnormalities. A much more common cause of head enlargement is a familial large head, in which the growth line may cross centiles but the other signs and symptoms are usually absent.

An abnormally small head is known as microcephaly. This may arise from some abnormality of brain development in pregnancy, or may be a sign of impaired brain growth due to some peri- or postnatal insult. Very rarely, it is associated with craniostenosis (cranio-synostosis). Usually this condition results in an abnormally shaped head. A small but normally shaped head results only from total craniostenosis which is extremely rare and is usually associated with other symptoms and signs.

Microcephaly cannot be defined by any absolute cut-off point. Head measurements well below the second centile are compatible with normal intellect. The probability of abnormality is higher if the measurement is below the −2.67SD line (0.4 centile). Some ethnic groups tend to have small head measurements, and the use of growth charts not designed for them can be misleading.

Early recognition of craniostenosis is important and should be included in teaching programmes; it is not necessarily detected by routine measurement of the head circumference.

Early treatment for hydrocephalus is desirable, although there is no conclusive evidence that it improves outcome. There is no specific treatment for microcephaly.

Recommendations for head circumference measurement

- The head circumference should be recorded **before discharge from hospital** following birth. This is an important measurement and should be performed and recorded carefully. If there is excessive oedema or moulding of the scalp following birth, this should also be recorded and if possible the measurement should be repeated a few days later.

- Head measurement should subsequently be undertaken at approximately **6–8 weeks of age**. It should be plotted on the chart and also written in figures. If there is no concern at this time, no further routine measurements are needed, but the head circumference should always be measured and recorded if there is any concern about a baby's growth, health, or development.

- If the growth line is **crossing centiles upwards,** and the child shows symptoms or signs compatible with hydrocephalus or other abnormality, urgent specialist opinion is essential. If there are no accompanying symptoms or signs, two measurements over a 4-week period are acceptable. Beyond this time limit, a decision must be made either to accept the situation as normal or to refer the child immediately for specialist examination.

- There is **no** justification for repeated measurements spread over many months, a practice which is to be deplored because it creates excessive anxiety. Modern imaging techniques make it simple to obtain a definitive diagnosis at an early stage.

- A head measurement above or below the 2.67SD line (99.6 centile and 0.4 centile respectively) at any stage is an indication for **more detailed assessment**. A small or a large head may be a reflection of genetic characteristics, and the parents' head measurements should always be checked. If they are in keeping with that of the baby and the baby appears to be developing normally, referral may not be necessary.

- If the growth line **crosses centiles downwards** but the baby is otherwise well and thriving, no special arrangements need be made. Concern should be expressed to the parents only if it becomes clear that the growth line is not only below the second centile but is also falling away from it.

- These apparently straightforward monitoring procedures must **not** be regarded as simple screening tests. **Skill and judgement** are required in deciding how to interpret the measurements, and no single pass–fail criterion can be proposed.

Research

Although these guidelines are generally accepted, little is known about the accuracy, value, or optimal timing of regular head circumference measurement or the relative merits of different referral criteria.

Appendix: Regression to the mean*

Charts of weight attained, also known as weight distance charts, are derived from cross-sectional data, and they allow weight to be expressed as a centile relative to the reference population, adjusted for age and sex. Such charts are also used to monitor weight velocity, on the grounds that a normally growing infant stays close to his or her chosen weight centile. This means that weight faltering is often inferred from the infant's weight falling across centiles. However, weight distance centiles should not be used in this way, as they are derived from cross-sectional data and cannot quantify changes in weight.

Over a period of time, infant weight tends to drift (or regress) towards the median—the tendency is to become less extreme with passing time. Thus an infant on the second weight centile is likely to show catch-up growth, whereas 98th centile infants tend on average to catch down. A weight velocity reference that compensates for regression to the mean is called a conditional reference. It answers the question: 'Knowing the infant's previous weight, what is her likely weight now?'

* Reproduced with permission of the BMJ Publishing Group from Cole, T.J. (1995). Conditional reference charts to assess weight gain in British infants. *Archives of Disease in Childhood* 73, 8–16.

The concept of regression to the mean is a statistical phenomenon. It states that if individuals or groups of individuals are weighed once, and later weighed again, their weight centile on the second occasion tends, on average, to be nearer the median than on the first occasion. This may seem counter-intuitive—surely an infant on, say, the second weight centile ought on average to stay there rather than move to a higher centile?

This phenomenon is about averages—it does not say that *every* infant on the second centile will catch up, only that a majority will. To see why, consider a randomly selected child at, say, 12 months of age. Knowing nothing about her we expect her to be average for her age, with an expected weight on the population median. Now imagine that we are given the information that her weight at 9 months was on the second centile. How should this extra knowledge alter our expectation of her weight at 12 months? The fact that she was below the median 3 months earlier obviously means that she ought still to be below the median, but by how much?

There is a range of possibilities. At one extreme, if weight tracks perfectly between 9 and 12 months, then we should expect her to remain on the second centile. Conversely, if there is no tracking at all between the two ages, our initial expectation will be unaltered, and we should still expect her to be on the median at 12 months. Thus the alternatives range from the second to the 50th centile, depending on how strongly weight tracks between 9 and 12 months. (Her *actual* centile at 12 months may well be below the second centile, but her average or expected centile will be above it.)

In this context tracking is synonymous with correlation, and perfect tracking requires perfect correlation. This is impossible, and so the extreme case of expecting her to remain on the second centile is ruled out. Her predicted weight centile at 12 months has to be above the second centile—less extreme than her weight centile at 9 months—and so her weight appears to regress towards the median. The same argument, in the reverse direction, applies to infants with weight centiles above the median.

The amount of regression to the mean depends on how highly correlated weights are at the two ages, and so the way to adjust for regression to the mean is to quantify this correlation.

Notes and references

A more extensive bibliography is available on growth disorders and growth monitoring; see p. xi for details.

1. Ghosh, S. (1993). Second thoughts on growth monitoring. *Indian Pediatrics* 30, 449–53. (Contains a useful bibliography on GM in developing countries.)
2. Barker, D.J., Gluckman, P.D., Godfrey, K.M., Harding, J.E., Owens, J.A., and Robinson, J.S. (1993). Fetal nutrition and cardiovascular disease in adult life. *Lancet* 341, 938–41.
3. Useful papers on failure to thrive include Cole, T.J. (1995). Conditional reference charts to assess weight gain in British infants. *Archives of Disease in Childhood* 73, 8–16. Wright, C.M., Matthews, J.N., Waterston, A., and Aynsley-Green, A. (1994). What is a normal rate of weight gain in infancy? *Acta Paediatrica* 83, 351–6; Puckering, C., Pickles, A., Skuse, D., Heptinstall, E., Dowdney, L., and Zur-Spiro, S. (1995). Mother–child interaction and the cognitive and behavioural development of four year old children with poor growth. *Journal of Child Psychology and Psychiatry* 36, 573–96 (this is an important paper as it describes a whole cohort of children with poor growth rather than a selected series.
4. The *Journal of Medical Screening* (1995) is publishing a symposium on growth monitoring, including papers on reliability and accuracy, psychological aspects and public health value of GM. See also Betts, P.R., Voss, L.D., and Bailey, B.J. (1992). Measuring the heights of very young children. *British Medical Journal* 304, 1351–52.
5. Height monitoring programmes are discussed in several papers: e.g. Ahmed, M.L., Allen, A.D., Sharma, A., Macfarlane, J.A., and Dunger, D.B. (1993). Evaluation of a district growth screening programme: the Oxford Growth Study. *Archives of Disease in Childhood* 69, 361–5; Voss, L.D., Mulligan, J., Betts, P.R., and Wilin, T.J. (1992). Poor growth in school entrants as an index of organic disease: the Wessex growth study. *British Medical Journal* 305, 1400–2; Lindsay, R., Feldkamp, M., Haris, D., Robertson, J., and Rallison, M. (1994). Utah Growth Study: growth standards and the prevalence of growth hormone deficiency. *Journal of Pediatrics* 125, 29–35.
6. Cole, T.J. (1994). Do growth chart centiles need a face lift? *British Medical Journal* 308, 641–2. (Describes the rationale for the new growth charts.)
   Freeman, J.V., Cole, T.J., Chinn, S., Jones, P.R.M., White, E.M., and Preece, M.A. (1995). Cross sectional stature and weight reference curves for the UK, 1990. *Archives of Disease in Childhood* 73, 17–24. (Provides the data on which the new charts are based.)
7. Cole, T.J., Freeman, J.V., and Preece, M.A. (1995). Body mass index reference curves for the UK, 1990. *Archives of Disease in Childhood*, 75, 25–9.
8. See Hindmarsh, P., Hulse, J.A., and Schilg, S. (1996) *British Medical Journal*, 312, for debate on these proposals. Work in preparation (Cole, T.J.) suggests their impact is heavily dependent on the extent of the measurement error.

8

Laboratory and radiological screening tests

This chapter covers:
Phenylketonuria and hypothyroidism (including thyroid disorders in Down's syndrome)
Other metabolic disorders
Cystic fibrosis
Duchenne muscular dystrophy
Urine analysis and urine infections: reflux
Haemoglobinopathies
Liver disease in infancy
Hypercholesterolaemia
Atlanto-axial subluxation in Down's syndrome
Lead poisoning
Neuroblastoma and coeliac disease

In general, screening procedures requiring laboratory or radiological tests have been subjected to more critical evaluation than clinical examinations, presumably because of the obvious costs involved and the requirements for careful organization.

We have not undertaken a detailed critical review of those programmes which are run on a nationwide basis, since they have in general been planned and managed by groups with a combined expertise not available to the present Working Party.* However, the question of screening for iron deficiency has been considered in detail and is the subject of a separate chapter.

Phenylketonuria and Congenital Hypothyroidism

Screening programmes for phenylketonuria (PKU) and congenital hypothyroidism (CH) are well-established. Their value is now accepted and although they are expensive they are thought to be cost-effective. The results of the PKU programme are good if care is coordinated by

* The Department of Health has commissioned reviews of some aspects of laboratory screening and these are expected to be available early in 1996.

expert clinicians and dietitians. Age at the start of treatment and quality of phenylalanine control in the first few years of life are important determinants of psychological outcome. Rapid referral of infants with positive screening tests to a specialist unit is therefore mandatory.

The benefits of CH screening are worthwhile but are less impressive than in the case of PKU. The level of thyroid-stimulating hormone (TSH) at the time of diagnosis, which is an indicator of the severity of hypothyroidism, is an important prognostic marker, suggesting that in severe cases the impairment of neurological development is not fully reversible.

Importance of audit, monitoring and feedback

The organization of screening for PKU and CH is currently under investigation and a national audit is being undertaken. Maintenance of a register of cases is important and must not be neglected in the re-organized NHS.

It is vital to ensure continuing laboratory quality control, very high coverage, and prompt follow-up of positive screening tests. Litigation costs for 'missed' cases are already considerable and will rise inexorably. Audit reveals that there are several reasons why coverage may fall short of 100 per cent; these include long stays in neonatal intensive care units, homelessness, travelling families, etc.[1]

Careful monitoring and clear accountability are essential if disasters are to be avoided, since the programme involves many different staff and procedures: blood sampling by midwives, processing of results by community child health departments, repeat tests by health visitors, and referrals arranged through general practitioners.

Parents must be informed about the tests; this may involve both written information (in the personal child health record) and verbal explanation. They should be given the results—it is not safe for parents or professionals to assume that the result is normal unless they hear otherwise.

It may never be possible to screen 100 per cent of the population and no laboratory test can ever be totally reliable. The diagnoses of PKU and CH should always be considered in appropriate clinical circumstances, and there should be no hesitation in repeating the investigations whenever there is doubt. This is particularly important in the case of CH since, for a variety of reasons, the screening procedure misses a few cases.[2]

Hypothyroidism in Down's syndrome

Individuals with Down's syndrome have a marked increase in the incidence of *biochemical* hypothyroidism and a smaller increase in hyperthyroidism.[3] About 15 per cent of adolescents with Down's syndrome are hypothyroid. The clinical diagnosis of hypothyroidism is difficult in these children as the features are similar to those of Down's syndrome itself. The aetiology is heterogeneous, but an autoimmune thyroiditis is often responsible. Neither the presence of microsomal antibodies nor the finding of high TSH levels necessarily imply clinical thyroid dysfunction, but these features may be an indication to check thyroxine levels more frequently.

A case can be made for routine screening, but there is no generally agreed screening programme for this problem. The Down's Syndrome Association recommends that as a minimum every child should have thyroxine, TSH, and thyroid antibody levels measured at least once before their fifth birthday and every 3 years thereafter. This guideline should be evaluated to determine how often and how effectively it identifies a child who would have been missed by informal observation or growth monitoring.

Other inherited metabolic disorders

Screening for many other disorders is possible and is undertaken in some parts of the UK* and in several other countries. Examples of conditions whose early detection may be both useful and cost effective are galactosaemia, maple syrup urine disease, homocystinuria, medium-chain acylCoA dehydrogenase deficiency, and biotinidase deficiency.

Cystic fibrosis

Screening for cystic fibrosis in the neonatal period is not regarded as a routine programme, but is available in some regions. This permits very early detection so that treatment can begin before lung damage occurs. Early diagnosis may be valued by parents, but there is as yet no clear evidence of objective benefit.

* In Scotland the Guthrie test includes testing for galactosaemia and anonymized HIV testing. Some regions in England carry out anonymized surveillance for maternal HIV.

Muscular dystrophy

It is technically possible to screen all boys for Duchenne muscular dystrophy at birth and some authorities have advocated this. The advantage of early diagnosis would be that the birth of further affected boys could be avoided. The main argument against this procedure has been that the total number of births thus prevented would be very small, so that the procedure might not justify its cost. An alternative approach is to screen all boys who first walk later than 18 months (the third centile), since 50 per cent of cases are late walkers (conversely it can be calculated that between 0.5 and 1.0 per cent of late-walking boys have Duchenne muscular dystrophy). This proposal has not been widely adopted as a formal screening policy, although a high index of suspicion should be maintained in this situation.

Urine infections

Urine examination as a screening test

Screening for proteinuria and asymptomatic bacteriuria has been advocated in the past on the grounds that chronic pyelonephritis resulting in chronic renal failure might be a preventable condition. We could find no convincing evidence that this is a worthwhile procedure.

Management of urine infections

Primary care staff should be aware that urinary tract infection (UTI) is common in infants. UTI should be considered in any infant with an unexplained pyrexia of 38.5 or above and, if possible, a urine specimen should be obtained. Infants with a first UTI should be referred for investigation.[4]

Vesico-ureteric reflux has an important association with urinary infections and there is a familial predisposition. It has been suggested that the siblings or children of any individual with this condition should undergo a micturating cystogram to ensure early identification. The implications of this policy need further evaluation.

The complex issues raised by antenatal ultrasound screening for urinary tract anomalies are outside the scope of this report.

Screening for haemoglobinopathies

The two most important haemoglobinopathies are sickle cell disease (SCD) and the thalassaemias, although there are a number of other less common abnormal haemoglobins.[5]

Approximately 3.3 per cent of the total UK population belongs to a racial group with a significant risk of having an abnormal haemoglobin. One person in 80 of West African origin and 1 in 200 of Jamaican origin has sickle cell disease. There are said to be approximately 6000 people with SCD in the UK, and it is estimated that between 75 and 300 babies are born with the condition each year.

There is a significant morbidity and mortality from SCD, particularly in the first 3 years of life. Causes include impaired immunity and fulminating pneumococcal infection. The latter can be prevented by penicillin prophylaxis which needs to be started by 3 months of age. Pneumococcal vaccine may also be useful. Parents can be taught to recognize splenic sequestration crises.

In the UK there are an estimated 450 people with homozygous thalassaemia, mostly of beta type, and about 60 children are born each year with the condition. Children with thalassaemia usually present with anaemia and failure to thrive. These features should lead to early diagnosis, followed by treatment with blood transfusion and iron chelation therapy.

Screening programmes aim to reduce the morbidity and mortality rates of infants born with haemoglobinopathies. Antenatal screening and advice should be followed by counselling, fetal diagnosis and termination of affected pregnancies, if the parents so wish.

People with SCD often feel that their condition is poorly understood and that they do not receive the help they need when acutely ill. Screening for haemoglobinopathies should be undertaken in parallel with other improvements in the care offered to individuals with these conditions. It is a complex undertaking, involving health education and the primary health care team together with obstetric, haematological, genetic, and paediatric services. People with SCD may need practical help to improve quality of life, for example better housing to avoid cold damp conditions which may precipitate crises. Skilled counsellors are essential and there are some difficult ethical problems.

Screening should be universal in districts where the ethnic groups concerned make up more than 15 per cent of the antenatal clinic population. Selective screening may be appropriate if the proportion is lower. Such a service is likely to be cost effective provided that appropriate treatment is initiated as soon as the diagnosis is made. There is evidence that such a programme is acceptable to and well used by the ethnic groups involved.

Liver disease in infancy: extrahepatic biliary atresia

The incidence of clinically significant liver disease in infancy is at least 1 in 3000 births. Of these, about 1 in 5 have extrahepatic biliary atresia (EHBA). Early diagnosis of this condition is important because surgery (the Kasai operation) is more effective if it is carried out by 6 weeks of age. Other liver diseases (hepatitis, a_1-antitrypsin deficiency, galactosaemia, etc.) would also benefit from early diagnosis. In addition, the problem of bleeding due to vitamin K deficiency could be avoided.

There is no simple screening procedure for liver disease or EHBA.[6] The clinical features of these conditions include prolonged jaundice with yellow sclerae, a high conjugated ('direct') bilirubin, and in some cases hypoglycaemia. However, benign prolonged jaundice is much more common than liver disease; the incidence of jaundice persisting to 2 weeks of age is around 15 per cent and even at 4 weeks it is 2.6 per cent. Many of these infants are breastfed (so-called 'breast-milk jaundice').

Prolonged jaundice alone would, therefore, lack specificity as a screening test. The addition of other observations and tests, such as orange urine, pale stools, or urine bilirubin, might improve specificity, but such a programme has yet to be evaluated in practice.

Familial hypercholesterolaemia

This is a dominantly inherited disorder with an incidence of 0.1–0.2 per cent (1 in 500 to 1 in 1000). It carries a higher risk of early heart disease than does polygenic hypercholesterolaemia. It is not feasible at present to screen all children for this condition or for the other hyperlipidaemias. Screening and management of the relatives, including children, of any person suffering coronary heart disease at a young age (i.e. below 50 years of age for a male and below 60 for a female) remains controversial.[7]

Atlanto-axial instability in people with Down's syndrome

This condition is more common in females, and the overall rate has been variously reported at between 12 and 22 per cent. Rarely, it may be associated with cervical cord damage. It has been suggested that there is an increased risk of cord compression for those who participate in vigorous sports (particularly trampolining or high board diving), but there are very few cases in the world literature of injuries sustained during sporting activities. The risk appears to be higher following whiplash injury in road traffic accidents and other forms of trauma, and as a result of neck positioning during anaesthesia. In many cases the onset of cervical cord compression is insidious rather than acute, and can be identified by alteration in the gait and tendon reflexes.

Screening for atlanto-axial instability using radiographs of the spine to measure the atlanto-odontoid interval (AOI) has been recommended. The interpretation of these radiographs is often difficult, and the test–retest reliability is low unless the radiographs are taken under standardized conditions. Failure to do this has resulted in exaggerated estimates of the risks. There is no evidence that those with a genuinely increased AOI are at increased risk of dislocation or subluxation. For all these reasons, the consensus of opinion is against screening.[8]

Subclinical lead poisoning

There is a robust association between elevated lead levels in the blood and teeth and reduction in intellectual functioning. It is not clear whether the association is causal; the magnitude of the effect is small; and there is little indication that intervention in children with no other clinical evidence of lead intoxication is likely to be beneficial or cost effective. The American Academy of Pediatrics has proposed a screening programme for subclinical lead intoxication, but there has been little support for this in the UK.[9]

Other screening programmes

There have been proposals that screening should be undertaken for neuroblastoma and coeliac disease. The evidence to date does not support the introduction of either programme.

Recommendations

Phenylketonuria and hypothyroidism

- Purchasers should identify **one individual** to take an overview of these screening programmes and ensure that referral, investigation and management are well coordinated.
- Parents should know the reasons for doing these tests and should receive the results.

Thyroid disorders in Down's syndrome

- The programme of screening recommended by the Down's Syndrome Association should be introduced **on a trial basis** and audited.

Other inherited metabolic disorders, including cystic fibrosis and muscular dystrophy

At present we recommend only that a **high level of awareness** is maintained regarding the presenting features of these conditions. Suspect cases should be referred for the appropriate diagnostic tests without hesitation. Purchasers should be aware that DNA technology may greatly extend the feasibility of and demand for screening in the next few years.

Urine analysis as a screening test

- This is **not** recommended, but there should be a local policy regarding the referral and investigation of infants with urinary infections.

Further research is needed in this subject. There are practical difficulties in ensuring that all UTIs in infants are accurately diagnosed and appropriately investigated. The optimal approach to investigation of infants with a family history of reflux also needs further study.

Haemoglobinopathies

- The service for people with haemoglobinopathies **should be reviewed in each district** with a view to raising the standard of care and considering the introduction of a screening programme. Screening for these conditions cannot be considered in isolation.

Liver disease in infancy

- Primary care staff should be aware of the possible significance of **prolonged jaundice** and should not readily dismiss it on the assumption that it is caused by breast-milk. The finding of **pale stools and/or orange urine** (provided that the baby is not dehydrated) should heighten suspicion and is an indication for immediate specialist opinion.

- Some of the reported late diagnoses are due to delays in referral to specialist units. Paediatricians in turn should ensure that such babies are **investigated promptly** and, if conjugated hyperbilirubinaemia is found, consider referral to a **specialist centre.**

- Until further evidence is available, **no** formal screening programme can be recommended.

Familial hypercholesterolaemia

- Screening should be confined to the **families of known sufferers** from this condition.

Screening for atlanto-axial subluxation in Down's syndrome

- We do **not** recommend this and do not consider that the evidence justifies screening. The normal precautions for travel in cars and minibuses should be enforced. Anaesthetists should be aware of the possible hazards of neck hyperextension.

- The diagnosis should be considered in any individual with **symptoms and signs compatible with spinal cord compression.**

Subclinical lead intoxication

- Screening for elevated blood lead levels is **not** recommended.

Neuroblastoma and coeliac disease

- Screening for these conditions is **not** recommended.

Notes and references

1. Streetly, A., Grant, C., Bickler, G., Eldridge, P., Bird, S., and Griffiths, W. (1994). Variation in coverage by ethnic group of neonatal (Guthrie) screening programme in south London. *British Medical Journal* 309, 373–4.
2. Grant, D.B. (1995). Congenital hypothyroidism: optimal management in the light of 15 years' experience of screening. *Archives of Disease in Childhood* 72, 85–9.
3. Selikowitz, M. (1993). A five-year longitudinal study of thyroid function in children with Down syndrome. *Developmental Medicine and Child Neurology* 35, 396–401. (For further information, contact the Down's Syndrome Association.)
4. Ansari, B.M., Jewkes, F., and Davies, S.G. (1995). Urinary tract infection in children. Part I: Epidemiology, natural history, diagnosis and management. *Journal of Infection* 30, 3–6.
   Wettergren, B. and Jodal, U. (1995). Spontaneous clearance of asymptomatic bacteriuria in infants. *Acta Paediatrica Scandinavica* 79, 300–4.
   Pead, L. and Maskell, R. (1994). Study of urinary tract infection in children in one health district. *British Medical Journal* 309, 631–4.
5. For a comprehensive review see *Sickle cell, thalassaemia and other haemoglobinopathies: report of a Working Party of the Standing Medical Advisory Committee.* HMSO, London (1993).
6. Mowat, A.P., Davidson, L.L., and Dick, M.C. (1995). Earlier identification of biliary atresia and hepatobiliary disease: selective screening in the third week of life. *Archives of Disease in Childhood* 72, 90–2.
7. Primrose, E.D., Savage, J.M., Boreham, C.A., Cran, G.W., and Strain, J.J. (1994). Cholesterol screening and family history of vascular disease. *Archives of Disease in Childhood* 71, 239–42.
8. Morton, R.E., Ali Kahn, M., Murray-Leslie, C., and Elliott, S. (1995). Atlantoaxial instability in Down's syndrome: a five year follow up study. *Archives of Disease in Childhood* 72, 115–19. *Commentary*, Chapman, S. pp. 118–19.
9. Harvey, B. (1994). Should blood lead screening recommendations be revised? *Pediatrics* 93, 201–4 (for USA view).
   Pocock, S.J., Smith, M., and Baghurst, P. (1994). Environmental lead and children's intelligence: a systematic review of the epidemiological evidence. *British Medical Journal* 309, 1189–97 (for UK view).

9

Iron deficiency

This chapter:
- defines iron deficiency
- describes its effects
- discusses screening and primary prevention
- outlines recommendations

Definition

Iron deficiency anaemia (IDA) is defined in early childhood by a haemoglobin (Hb) level of less than 11 g/dl together with other evidence of iron deficiency and a response to iron administration. Iron deficiency is not necessarily accompanied by anaemia. It can be defined by a transferrin saturation of less than 16 per cent, a serum iron of less than 14 µmol/l, or a serum ferritin of less than 10 mcg/l. Zinc protoporphyrin (ZPP) levels have also been used to define iron deficiency. ZPP increases when erythropoiesis is ineffective, as in iron deficiency states, and a ZPP level of greater than 50 µmol per mol haem is suggestive of iron deficiency (although this may also occur in other disorders).

The predisposing factors and causes of iron deficiency include: inadequate dietary intake of iron, often in association with drinking unmodified cow's milk ('doorstep' milk), prematurity and low birth-weight, and use of foodstuffs and beverages (notably tea) which reduce the availability of iron for absorption. Unmodified cow's milk increases intestinal blood loss, although the significance of this is uncertain.

Effects

Iron deficiency anaemia is associated with deficits in a variety of developmental and behavioural measures,[1] typically of between 10 and 15 points on standard tests such as the Bayley test. These deficits are probably due to a direct effect on the brain rather than being a result of anaemia. The behavioural and intellectual deficits are reversible with iron therapy and, in view of the lower prevalence of IDA in older children, are assumed to recover spontaneously in many cases as the child's diet becomes more varied.

Long-term follow-up of children who have recovered from IDA shows some small persisting intellectual deficits, but these may reflect the adverse environment which caused the iron deficiency and should not be interpreted as conclusive evidence of irreversible impairment of brain development. Nevertheless, it seems undesirable for young children to suffer easily treatable nutritional deficits which might affect their developmental progress.

Prevalence

IDA is a common disorder in preschool children (Table 9.1). Various studies suggest a prevalence in the UK of between 5 and 40 per cent. It is thought to be more common in the underprivileged and in ethnic minorities, but in the population as a whole the correlation with socio-economic status is weak and it is by no means rare in the better-off. Less information is available about school-aged children, but the prevalence appears to vary between 3 and 10 per cent.

Screening

A strong case has been made for the introduction of screening programmes for IDA, particularly in areas of poverty. Screening is acceptable to and popular with parents, the screening test appears to be simple and cheap, and an effective treatment is available.

Table 9.1   Iron deficiency and anaemia*

Measurement	Prevalence (%)		
	1½–2½ years	2½–3½ years	3½–4½ years
Hb < 11 g/dl	12	6	6
Hb < 10 g/dl	2	1	0
Ferritin < 10 mcg/l	28	18	15
Ferritin < 5 mcg/l	9	3	3

* Based on a nationally representative sample
Source: Gregory, J.R., Collins, D.L., Davies, P.S.W., Hughes, J.M. and Clarke, P.C. *National diet and nutrition survey: children ages 1½ to 4½ years*. London, HMSO, 1995.

Nevertheless, there are some arguments against screening:

1. The test requires a blood sample which to some parents might be seen as an unnecessary intrusion.

2. Although haemoglobinometers are simple to use, meticulous technique in collecting the sample and using the instrument are essential, particularly when screening for IDA is based solely on the Hb level. The instruments available to primary care teams have a higher measurement error than those used in laboratories, and little is known about the sensitivity, specificity, and positive predictive value of Hb measurements carried out in the primary care setting. Severe IDA would probably be identified without difficulty, but detection of the mild cases who would form the bulk of the screen-positive children might be less reliable.

3. The timing of the screening test presents problems. Iron intake probably falls to a level below the daily requirement in the second half of the first year in many at-risk children, but the child does not necessarily show biochemical evidence of iron deficiency or develop anaemia until considerably later. Thus many children who would pass the screening test at the age of 12 or 18 months become iron deficient in the third year. Conversely, some children who are iron deficient in the second year undoubtedly recover as they eat a more varied diet in the third and fourth years of life. There is so far no clear evidence on the optimal age or ages for screening, although clearly it would be desirable to carry out any screening test in association with other routine child health surveillance checks.

4. The identification of children who are iron deficient but have not yet developed anaemia could be facilitated by the use of other tests in addition to Hb, but this would complicate the procedure and increase costs. Some of the recommended tests would require a venepuncture rather than a capillary specimen.

5. Iron deficiency is potentially preventable, and resources should be devoted to primary prevention rather than screening (which is secondary prevention).

Primary prevention

In theory primary prevention could be achieved by the following measures.

1. Provision of iron supplements for premature and low birth-weight infants; this is now standard practice.

2. Not using unmodified ('doorstep') cow's milk in the first year of life as the child's main milk drink (it is not necessary to eliminate it altogether). NB Although breast milk has a low iron concentration the bioavailability is very high.

3. Not giving young children tea.

4. Continued use of infant formula or follow-on milks in the second half of the first year of life.

5. Weaning on to mixed feeding by 6 months of age.

6. Iron supplementation for *all* infants has been suggested and is the usual practice in some countries.

Nutrition education may reduce the incidence of IDA in some circumstances, but the impact appears to be variable and in some situations minimal. It must depend on a complex interaction between biological, cultural, and social factors.

The use of iron-fortified formula or follow-on milks reduces the incidence of IDA, although the higher cost compared with doorstep milk is a problem for some parents. We are not aware of any direct comparison of standard and follow-on formula in the UK. A Canadian trial showed follow-on formula to be superior in preventing iron deficiency, but the level of iron in the standard 'comparison' formula was much lower than is usual in Europe.[2]

The universal prescription of iron supplementation is routine in some countries and reduces the incidence of IDA substantially but has some disadvantages.

1. Some infants are reluctant to take iron medicine and this may cause feeding conflicts with the parent.

2. Iron in overdose is dangerous, and it is undesirable to keep hazardous medicines in homes with young children unless absolutely necessary.

3. It has been suggested that iron treatment may increase the risk of infection and also may affect growth adversely.

4. Iron treatment could in theory increase iron overload in a child with undiagnosed thalassaemia. However, most cases of thalassaemia have presented before the age at which IDA becomes a common concern.

Recommendations

- All parents should be **informed** about the advantages of iron-fortified formula feeding over doorstep milk, and the use of doorstep milk as the main drink should be **discouraged**, at least until the first birthday.

- Universal screening for IDA across the whole of the UK is **not** recommended.

- All members of the primary health care team should be aware of the **high incidence of IDA.**

- The Hb should be checked in any infant **whose diet is causing concern.** This can best be achieved by ensuring easy access to a haemoglobinometer in the primary care setting, but those who use it must be familiar with the technique and interpretation.

- Efforts at **primary prevention** should be intensified. However, advice on good nutrition for young children should not be given in isolation, but should be part of a wider programme of support, particulary for vulnerable families who need extra support (p. 51).

- The advice of a **dietician** familiar with the dietary customs of other ethnic groups and cultures should be available to the primary health care team.

- **Iron supplementation for premature and low birth-weight** (small for gestational age) infants should be given.

- Universal iron supplements are **not** recommended. A 4–6 week course of iron therapy[3] should be given to any infant whose Hb is below 11 g/dl unless there is any other obvious explanation, and the Hb should then be rechecked.

- Any infant whose **Hb is below 7.5** should also have a full blood count and an assessment of iron status and, if thought to be indicated by the laboratory, thalassaemia and sickle cell disease should be excluded. The laboratory should advise the primary health care team on the interpretation of the results. (NB It can be difficult to exclude thalassaemia trait in children with iron deficiency, but it is doubtful whether this is necessary if the Hb level responds to iron, since the diagnosis is of no relevance in infancy or childhood.)

- In districts or localities where there is severe socio-economic deprivation and a substantial proportion of ethnic minority families, **existing**

screening programmes should be continued provided that they are adequately monitored, are shown to be reaching the most at risk members of the community, and are accompanied by continuing efforts at primary prevention.

• We do **not** think that the evidence supports the extension of whole-population screening programmes at present, *except* as a means of measuring the effectiveness of intensified efforts at primary prevention in a carefully planned project.

Research needs

It is still not clear why some infants become iron deficient while others do not. Dietary variables do not seem to be the complete explanation. Differences in weaning practices, temperamental differences in the readiness of infants to eat new foods, variations in iron stores earlier in infancy, and individual differences in the absorptive capacity for iron may all play a part.

The apparent lack of effectiveness of health education measures in changing feeding practices needs further study.

Although the short-term impact of IDA on development seems to be beyond question in early infancy and in toddlers, less is known about these effects in older children or teenagers.

Notes and references

A more extensive bibliography is available on iron deficiency; see p. xi for details.

1. The following articles give an overview of the subject:
   Lozoff, B. (1994). Iron deficiency and infant development. *Journal of Pediatrics* 125, 577–8; Oski, F.A. (1993); Iron deficiency in infancy and childhood. *New England Journal of Medicine* 329, 190–3. Pollitt, E. (1993). Iron deficiency and cognitive function. *Annual Reviews of Nutrition* 13, 521–37.
2. Moffatt, M.E.K., Longstaffe, S., Besant, J., and Dureski, C. (1994). Prevention of iron deficiency and psychomotor decline in high-risk infants through use of iron-fortified infant formula: a randomized clinical trial. *Journal of Pediatrics* 125, 527–34.
3. The dose should be 5 mg/kg/day of elemental iron.

10

Screening for hearing defects

This chapter:
- describes and defines hearing loss
- summarizes the epidemiology
- describes the impact of hearing loss on development
- lists and discusses the various approaches to screening
- makes recommendations for practice, monitoring, and research

The nature of hearing impairment

Hearing impairment is of two main types: sensorineural hearing loss (SNHL) and conductive hearing loss. The epidemiology[1] and causes are summarized in Table 10.1.

Sensorineural hearing loss

SNHL is caused by a lesion in the cochlea or the auditory nerve and its central connections. It may be unilateral or bilateral. Important causes and risk factors are summarized in Table 10.1.

In the absence of appropriate intervention children with SNHL suffer impairment of language acquisition. Educational difficulties follow and lead in turn to social isolation, an increased risk of mental health problems, and reduced prospects for independence in adult life. Intervention with amplification or cochlear implants and appropriate teaching help the child to acquire a means of communication by speech, signing, or both.

Conductive hearing loss

Conductive hearing loss is related to middle-ear pathology. In developed countries this is usually due to secretory otitis media, now more commonly known as otitis media with effusion (OME). In poorer communities there may be chronic suppurative otitis media with discharge and perforation. SNHL and middle-ear disease may coexist.

Table 10.1 Epidemiology, risk factors, and causes of hearing loss

- The estimated birth prevalence of congenital sensorineural or mixed hearing impairment (> 40 dBHL in the better ear averaged over the frequencies 0.5, 1, 2 and 4 kHz) is 1.16 per 1000.

- 1.3 per 1000 children have this degree of hearing loss and require a hearing aid; the difference is accounted for by acquired and conductive hearing loss

- Meningitis is the most important cause of acquired hearing loss and accounts for up to a fifth of profound hearing loss, though this figure may have fallen since the introduction of Hib vaccine and the consequent fall in the incidence of haemophilus meningitis.

- Ascertainment of less severe hearing loss in preschool children is incomplete, but at least 0.3 per 1000 have a hearing loss which, though less than 40 dB, is clinically significant and requires a hearing aid

- The incidence of SNHL is at least 10 times higher in babies admitted to neonatal intensive care units (NICU), compared with the 'normal' population. There are a number of risk factors including low birth-weight, gestational age below 32 weeks, prolonged ventilation, prolonged jaundice, ototoxic drugs, hypoxic ischaemic encephalopathy, neonatal meningitis, etc. NICU stay of more than 48 hours defines the at risk population more simply, though some babies who do not have a significantly increased risk of SNHL will then be tested unnecessarily. A substantial proportion (over half in some series) of NICU babies with SNHL have other disabilities as well

- Other factors which increase the risk of hearing loss include congenital infections (rubella, cytomegalovirus), dysmorphic syndromes, particularly those affecting the head and neck, family history of a close relative who needed a hearing aid before the age of 5 years, acute bacterial or tuberculous meningitis, and mumps (usually unilateral)

- If all high-risk factors are considered, between 40% and 70% of all cases could be identified by testing between 5% and 10% of all babies. This yield can only be obtained by a systematic and well-organized approach to the identification and testing of at-risk babies.

- Conductive hearing loss is extremely common. At least half of all preschool children have one or more episodes of OME. A much smaller number of children, perhaps around 7 per cent, have OME for at least half of the time between 2 and 4 years (see Fig. 10.1)

Parental smoking is a risk factor for OME. Breast-feeding may be protective. The role of allergy is uncertain. Some children are at particular risk of developing persistent OME. This group includes those with Down's syndrome, cleft palate, Turner's syndrome, and facial malformation syndromes.

The extent of the *disability* caused by OME is still controversial. Few research studies have differentiated between those children with transient

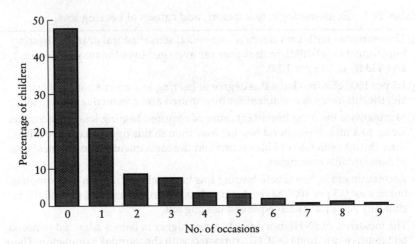

Fig. 10.1   Persistence diagram of OME. The definition of OME was bilateral flat tympanograms, indicating fluid in both ears. Over 1000 children were tested on nine occasions at 3-month intervals. In 69 per cent of cases, OME either did not occur or was transient. In 7.3 per cent of cases, OME was present for at least half the study period. There is as yet no way of identifying the group with prolonged OME except by serial testing of all children (at least four times), and therefore no feasible screening programme which could select this high-risk group. The solution is (a) to find markers which will indicate persistence of OME without the need to test every child serially or (b) to focus on the disability caused by OME (clinically evident hearing impairment, language delay, or unexplained behavioural problems). Solution (a) is preferable as it would offer the possibility of primary prevention; solution (b) is the only option available at present.
Based on Nijmegen cohort, date reworked by Stephenson *et al*, presented and discussed by Haggard. Acknowledgments to authors and Nuffield Hospitals Trust[4].

OME and minor hearing impairment, and those with persistent disease and more marked hearing loss. In addition, it is highly likely that hearing loss interacts with other factors, such as environmental deprivation, temperament, and genetic influences on the rate of language acquisition. Unilateral or asymmetric hearing loss may cause deficits in the ability to localize sound and to distinguish important sounds such as speech from background noise.

In those children with occasional self-limiting episodes, OME probably has a minimal influence on speech and language development, but severe persistent OME may result in significant delay in language acquisition, behaviour disturbance, and in some cases temporary balance disturbance.

Treatment

Surgery to ventilate the middle ear is effective while grommets remain patent, and this may be important for the child at a time of rapid language acquisition. The long-term benefits are much less certain. Conservative management is advocated for the majority of children who are not severely affected. Decongestants are not effective. The value of antibiotic and steroid therapy is unproven. An alternative approach for the most severely affected children is the provision of a low-power hearing aid. Continued audiological and educational supervision is essential.

Simply explaining the nature of the problem to parents or teachers is often helpful. Once they understand that the child has a hearing loss, they can communicate more effectively. Written information about OME should be available. A copy of the child's test results or audiogram, with appropriate explanation, is reassuring.

Unilateral hearing loss

Unilateral hearing loss is generally assumed to be primarily a social disadvantage in school, but it has been suggested that there may be subtle yet significant effects on cognitive development. It does not seem likely that these are sufficiently important to influence screening policy, but further research is needed.

Early diagnosis and intervention

There are several reasons for the current professional commitment to early diagnosis of congenital sensorineural hearing loss (CSNHL).

The reason most commonly quoted is that very early diagnosis might improve the outcome in terms of speech and language quality and communicative skill. Since age of diagnosis and intervention depend on so many factors, confirmation of this is very difficult to obtain and the results of published surveys are contradictory. However, it is clear that delayed diagnosis is not incompatible with good language acquisition and that family factors (social and communicative skills, attitudes, etc.) are an important determinant of outcome. The potential benefits of early intervention are unlikely to be realized unless families receive good support and counselling as well as guidance on amplification and communication.

Animal studies suggest that there is a sensitive or critical period for learning. Brain plasticity is greatest early in life, and meaningful sound input may be necessary to facilitate the development of neural connections. Nevertheless, in animal models significant cortical reorganization following cochlear lesions is possible even in adults. The excellent results obtained after cochlear implantation in children up to the age of 10 years also suggest that in humans the critical or sensitive period must last for several years. Thus, the question is not yet finally resolved, and the evidence that early intervention improves outcome is still equivocal. However, there are several other excellent reasons why screening may be useful:

- It is easier to achieve high coverage for screening and early detection services for babies in the first year of life than at any time subsequently until school entry.
- Most parents welcome early diagnosis of disabling conditions and have a low opinion of services which fail to identify serious long-term problems in their children.
- It is easier to establish the cause of CSNHL if it is diagnosed early. In particular, intrauterine infections become increasingly difficult or impossible to diagnose after the first few months of life.

Views of the deaf community

Deaf children of deaf parents are a special case. The aim of early diagnosis is to improve oral communication, but the strong views of some members of the deaf community on signing should be remembered and respected. It should not be assumed that all hearing impaired parents will unreservedly welcome early screening for their infants.

Arguments in favour of screening

Parents sometimes recognize severe hearing loss themselves, but hearing loss of moderate degree, or predominantly affecting high frequencies, is easily missed, sometimes for several years. Therefore a good case can be made for screening.

Since most cases of significant SNHL are congenital and the process of language acquisition begins at birth, the obvious time to screen is in the neonatal period. However, even universal neonatal screening would not detect all children with hearing loss for the following reasons:

1. SNHL due to congenital rubella and cytomegalovirus may deteriorate during the first 2 years of life, but may not be readily detectable in the neonatal period.

2. Some types of genetically determined SNHL are progressive and may present at any time in childhood. Until recently it has been thought that this applied only to a very small proportion of cases, but follow-up of large cohorts who had been shown to have normal hearing in the neonatal period suggests that hearing loss with an onset in the first year of life may be rather more common, perhaps at least 10–15 per cent.

Are there any disadvantages to screening?

In studies on universal neonatal screening, a small percentage of parents refuse the offer of a screening test. Some parents would prefer to put off the moment of diagnosis, and some may actively avoid it. The psychological reasons for this behaviour are probably complex and need further study. They might represent protection of self or partner against intolerable stress in the face of other life problems. It is clear that sensitivity to parental feelings is important. A screening test which seems routine to staff might be a major life event for the parent if the child turns out to have a hearing loss.

Approaches to screening

There are many possible strategies for screening for hearing loss[2] (Table 10.2).

Neonatal screening

*Universal neonatal screening** has attracted much attention[3] because it appears to offer access to a 'captive population' and it should be possible to achieve high coverage rates, but the rapid turnover and early discharge policy in most maternity units make this difficult in practice. The available methods are described in detail below. Currently, the most promising technique for universal screening is evoked otoacoustic emissions (EOAE) but there are still some unsolved problems with this method. The follow-up needed for babies who do not pass the screen

* The Minister of Health, John Bowis MP, has acknowledged the potential value of neonatal screening and a detailed report on the subject will be available in 1996.

Table 10.2 Summary of screening options in ascending order of estimated cost

---

No screening programme, reliance on parental recognition only

Active parental and professional education programme but no formal screening

Selective ('high risk') neonatal screening plus education programme

Distraction test at 6–9 months

Selective ('high risk') neonatal screening plus education programme plus distraction test at 6–9 months

Univeral neonatal screening plus education programme

Universal neonatal screening plus education programme plus distraction test at 6–9 months

---

(a) An education programme might include the use of information sheets (perhaps inserted in the personal child health record), questionnaires, videos, or parent interviews.

(b) In the present state of knowledge we do not think that any one option can confidently be described as the 'best buy'. The more expensive options are likely to detect more cases at an earlier stage, but the cost per case detected must rise steeply as well.

(c) The quality and supervision of the programme and the commitment of the staff are probably the most important factors in determining success.

increases both the cost and the amount of anxiety caused. These problems could to some extent be overcome if equipment becomes available for use in the home.

The main cost of universal neonatal screening is in personnel. The cost must be calculated in terms of the number of babies who can be tested in a typical week, not by dividing the time taken per test into the number of hours worked. Estimates of this figure vary from 30 or 35 to 80 babies per week (irrespective of the method used). It is probably lower in small units where the screeners cannot be kept fully occupied. The tasks of providing training for screeners, ensuring that all infants are tested (including those discharged from hospital early and those born at weekends or holidays, or at home), and maintaining standards present challenges which should not be underestimated.

Selective neonatal screening of high risk groups (Table 10.1) Case finding may be achieved via antenatal departments, neonatal intensive care units, postnatal wards, and the primary care team. The programme can be brought to parents' attention at antenatal classes and by devoting a page to hearing and risk factors in the personal child health record. Selective screening is increasingly popular and, as parents and professionals become more familiar with the concept of 'high risk', it is likely that demand for this service will become irresistible.

The methods used for neonatal screening The auditory response cradle (ARC) is an *automated behavioural method* which detects changes in the infant's head turns and bodily movements in response to a sound stimulus. This device was not designed, and is not suitable, for premature babies. Its sensitivity for the less severe degrees of SNHL is relatively low and it is unlikely to detect all cases with losses of 50 dB or greater, which is usually regarded as the desirable criterion for neonatal screening. In the past its reputation has suffered from difficulties with reliability and maintenance, although these have now been resolved. Notwithstanding the theoretical and practical concerns outlined above, satisfactory sensitivity and specificity have been reported and behavioural methods may have a role in universal screening.

Brain-stem evoked response audiometry (BSERA) involves the computer analysis of EEG signals evoked in response to a series of clicks. A full BSERA study is a skilled undertaking. Screening devices can be operated by unqualified staff after appropriate training and have been used for neonatal screening of high-risk babies, but this method is too time consuming for universal screening. Even in skilled hands, diagnostic BSERA testing may produce results which are difficult to interpret, particularly in NICU infants, and in some cases hearing loss has been incorrectly diagnosed. For this reason, audiologists are careful to confirm the diagnosis of CSNHL before fitting hearing aids.

Evoked otoacoustic emissions (EOAE) which are acoustic responses produced in the inner ear by the outer hair cells of the cochlea, and detected with a sensitive microphone placed in the ear canal. EOAE is a very sensitive test and detects hearing losses as low as 30 dBHL. In the Rhode Island study, for example, EOAE screening resulted in identification of 6 cases per 1000 births.

The test is easier and quicker than BSERA and is being used in several centres for universal screening. Unfortunately, there is a high failure rate in the first two days of life; around 60 per cent pass on day 1, 80 per cent on day 2 and over 95 per cent on subsequent days. Half are unilateral and half are bilateral failures. Ambient noise and technical difficulties may be partly responsible but can be overcome. Fluid in the middle ear and maturational delays are thought to be the main reasons for the high failure rate.

Those who have a normal response are regarded as passing the screen, although it is possible for an infant to have a 'normal' emission with a limited frequency range of normal hearing. The 'failures' undergo a second EOAE screening. All babies who fail the second

EOAE screen should then undergo BSERA, usually using the screening device (although in some centres these babies are referred directly for a diagnostic BSERA study).

Making use of parental observations

These can be enhanced by the use of a check list in the personal child health record, which alerts parents to the existence of hearing loss in babies and tells them what to look for. Parents are more likely to identify severe and profound hearing loss, and may easily overlook less severe or high frequency impairments.

Behavioural testing during the first year of life

This technique, which is known as the distraction test, requires two people working in collaboration. It depends on the infant's ability to turn and localize a sound source. A developmental maturity level of around 7 months is optimum for this test. Before this age, sitting balance, head control, and sound localization ability are imperfect. Beyond 10 months of age, the development of object permanence and increasing sociability make the test more difficult.

Prerequisites   Quiet conditions, proper equipment, adequate sound level monitoring, and careful technique are essential. The distraction technique is ideally suited for testing children around 6–9 months of age. Good results can be obtained if initial and regular refresher training courses are provided to ensure that technique is meticulous and standard guidelines are observed. Ideally, the test should be done in protected time, rather than during a busy baby clinic.

Hazards and problems of the distraction test   When inadequately performed, the distraction screening test is not merely valueless but can be positively harmful because the child's apparent responses to sound may persuade parents that their own worries about his or her hearing were unfounded. This can lead to delays in identification. The test may also be used, inappropriately in our view, to 'screen' babies with high risk factors such as a positive family history or a long stay in NICU. For several reasons such babies may be particularly difficult to test and should be referred for definitive diagnosis if this was not done in the neonatal period.

Many staff are still very committed to the distraction test and believe that it is valuable. It is possible that there is a publication bias and that districts whose results are satisfactory do not publish them. However, few of the published studies on the performance of this screening procedure under field conditions are encouraging. This is partly because few districts fulfil all the conditions set out in the previous paragraphs. Problems include the following:

- In practice, the sensitivity of the test is often low and many cases are missed. Poor test technique generates a large number of false positives. Coverage is often unsatisfactory, and the incidence of hearing loss is higher in non-attenders.
- Parents' concerns and important risk factors are ignored and inappropriate reassurance is given.
- The procedure, if properly performed, identifies many genuine but transient cases of hearing loss due to middle-ear disease. These rarely require treatment, but overload clinics and increase waiting times for definitive diagnosis for those children with more serious problems.

Dual pathology   Children can have both CSNHL and middle-ear disease. Sometimes the hearing impairment is attributed only to the middle-ear disease, and the child may be referred for ear, nose, and throat (ENT) management. Unless the hearing is rechecked at intervals, the sensorineural component of the hearing loss can easily be overlooked for many months.

Improving the distraction test   Costs can be reduced if the test is performed by one health visitor and one assistant. This can be done without any fall in standards. Reports are awaited on a new portable automated version of the distraction test (BeST) which can be operated by one person. It has also been suggested that the hearing level at which the baby 'passes' might be raised, since this would reduce the number of false-positive results while missing very few significant cases of SNHL. A system known as CAPAS is being used extensively in Holland.

Economic aspects   With increasing public awareness of hearing problems and high risk factors, many children (including most of those with risk factors) are diagnosed before the age at which the test is normally performed. If 40–50 per cent of all cases are found by a high-risk screening programme and parents identify a further proportion themselves, it is unlikely that the distraction test will detect more than a third of the total number of cases; a quarter or a fifth may be more realistic. Thus the 'incremental yield' (p. 86) will be relatively small and the cost per case detected correspondingly high.

There are two additional considerations. Firstly, any of the changes in the distraction test described above would, if shown to be practical, significantly alter the cost calculations. Secondly, the cost per case detected is greatly reduced if cases of OME discovered by screening are included in the 'yield'. However, this is not generally regarded as the function of the distraction test, for the reasons set out previously.

Testing between the ages of 18 and 42 months
In this age group it becomes possible to test hearing by methods involving cooperation.

Speech discrimination tasks, such as the McCormick Toy Test, require the child to respond by pointing to a series of objects named by the examiner in a very quiet voice. An automated version of the Toy Test is now available. These tests are enjoyed by children, and are easily learnt and applied accurately. Most children can perform them successfully by 39 months of age. At or beyond this age, inability to cooperate with the Toy Test is suggestive either of a hearing difficulty or some more general developmental problem.

The child may be required to give some *behavioural response* to measured sound produced either by voice or by a warbler or audiometer. These 'performance tests' are capable of giving accurate results if the tester is adequately trained, and are particularly useful when testing children whose first language is not English and with no staff available who speak the child's own language.

The more mature and cooperative child can be tested with headphones (*pure tone audiometry*).

We considered whether any further preschool screening test of hearing should be undertaken after the age of 7 months. This has been called an *'intermediate'* screen. The argument in favour is that a few children with acquired or progressive SNHL and those with severe OME may otherwise elude diagnosis until they start school, with possibly serious consequences for their learning and education. The disadvantages of such a policy are as follows:

1. The low yield of significant new cases.
2. The high incidence of transient OME.
3. The difficulty of determining which cases of OME are transient and

which are persistent (see Fig. 10.1). The ability to predict which cases would suffer some disability from their OME would be a useful advance, but as yet no such method is available.[4]

The school entry 'sweep' test of hearing
This test consists of a modified pure tone audiogram performed at fixed intensity level. Criteria for failure on this test vary from 20 through 25 to 30 dB at one or more frequencies and after one or two tests. Many variables affect the results of this procedure, including ambient noise, the skill of the screener, and the maturity of the child.

The school entrant 'sweep' test is used in most districts in the UK. Very few cases of severe SNHL remain undiagnosed at this age, except in children newly arrived in the UK, but occasionally a child is found to have a progressive hearing loss. A significant number of milder cases are detected and unilateral losses are usually identified for the first time. OME is very common and may have educational implications, even though few children require active treatment. Since the referral criteria and management of OME remain controversial and treatment resources are overstretched, each district and health board should define precisely its own policy and monitor the results.

Further screening tests of hearing after school entry appear to have a very small yield and we do not think that they can be justified. However, hearing should be assessed in any child experiencing learning, behavioural, or speech and language difficulties.

Impedance measurement
This is a technique for assessing middle-ear function and therefore of detecting fluid in the middle ear. It does not give a direct measure of hearing levels. It is a very sensitive test which detects even minor degrees of middle-ear dysfunction and is best reserved for use as a diagnostic procedure in specialist clinics. It should not be used as a primary screening procedure for preschool children. Although it has been suggested that school entrant screening might be improved by addition or substitution of impedance screening, this proposal has not undergone any extensive field testing.

Acquired hearing loss—meningitis
Early diagnosis reduces the incidence of most complications of acute bacterial meningitis. This may not invariably be true for sensorineural deafness, although steroids given at the start of antibiotic therapy may

reduce the risk of hearing loss. *All* young children who have had this condition should have an audiological assessment, even if they have been diagnosed early and have not been very ill.[5] Profound hearing loss following meningitis in a young child is an educational emergency, since the benefits to the child of having had previous experience of sound will be squandered if amplification and teaching are not provided promptly.

Recommendations

- **General comments** Across the country there is wide variation in the number of screening tests carried out, the referral policy, and the ease of access to treatment. Surprisingly few districts or health boards can provide data on the effectiveness of their programmes. Therefore there is still very little firm evidence on which to base our recommendations. Within the next few years, however, it should be possible to calculate the probable performance and cost of each of the options set out in Table 10.2.

- **Need for a well-organized audiology service** The first step in considering changes to the screening programme must be to examine the whole paediatric audiological service and to review present and future staffing needs. There is no point in creating an excellent screening network if the facilities for behavioural testing, definitive BSERA studies, ENT assessment, diagnosis, or education and rehabilitation are inadequate. All parents with hearing impaired children should have access to a centre with such facilities, and the need for paediatric, psychological, and genetic advice must be met.[6]

- **A systematic approach to increasing parental awareness about hearing loss, such as the use of a check list, should be adopted in all districts.** The full potential of this approach has yet to be adequately explored and evaluated, but there is sufficient professional support for us to recommend it as a matter of policy.

- **Parental suspicions about possible hearing loss must be taken seriously, and a rapid efficient referral route to an audiological centre must be available in *every* part of the country.** No parent who expresses concern about a child's hearing should be denied prompt referral to the audiological service.

- **'Intermediate' screening is not recommended.** However, it should be routine to ask the parents of preschool children whether they have any concerns about the child's hearing. An audiological assessment should be arranged for any child who has the following:

(a) significantly impaired language development;

(b) a history of chronic or repeated middle-ear disease or upper air-way obstruction;

(c) developmental or behavioural problems.

We emphasize that, whatever screening options are adopted in the first year of life, substantial numbers of children will need assessment in the 'intermediate' years. Most of these will have OME. A well-run clinical service can ensure that those few children who need surgical opinion or intervention are selected for referral to an ENT surgeon without creating long waiting lists. Children with conditions which put them at high risk of middle-ear disease should be assessed at regular intervals in a clinic with full diagnostic facilities including impedance equipment.

- **The school entry sweep test of hearing should be continued.** The diagnostic and referral pathway must be evaluated as well as the sweep test itself. After this, no further routine screening test of hearing is recommended.

- **Acquired hearing loss:** audiological assessment and follow-up should be arranged for any young child who has had bacterial meningitis, prolonged treatment with ototoxic drugs, or severe head injury, either before or soon after discharge from hospital.

- **Organization and equipment:** it is important that health authorities provide adequate conditions for hearing testing and that the staff involved have their own hearing tested every 2 years. All staff involved with screening tests of hearing should have access to the necessary equipment (sound-level meters, warble tone generators, etc.) and proper training in their use. Equipment should be checked and calibrated regularly.

- **Coordinator:** arrangements should be made in each district or health board for coordinating the local paediatric audiology programme, including screening, monitoring, training, and refresher courses (see also p. 214). Information should be collected on the coverage of screening programmes, the number of referrals, delays experienced between referral and diagnosis and between diagnosis and treatment, and the age at which each child with SNHL is diagnosed. Liaison with other disciplines and agencies is vital to ensure that nationally agreed standards of service are achieved and that the requirements of relevant legislation are fulfilled (p. 79).

- **Universal neonatal screening** is still largely a research procedure. We recommend that districts should begin to consider how they will respond if such a programme is shown to be the most cost-effective solution, but should not set up universal neonatal screening until the results of research in progress are known. Those centres with a well-organized universal screening programme and good data collection systems already in place should continue their present service. If they are also continuing their distraction test programme at 6–9 months, this should be monitored with particular care. We predict that this procedure will be found to be expensive in terms of cost per case detected in any district with an effective universal neonatal screening programme.

- **Selective or high risk screening** has much to commend it. The yield should be high and the cost relatively low.

- **The distraction test:** the future of this test has prompted considerable debate in recent years. We make the following suggestions:

  (a) Where *universal* neonatal screening is already in place, the advice given above should be followed.

  (b) Where there is an effective *selective* neonatal screen, a well-documented record of good results, and the ability to monitor the contribution of the distraction test continuously, the issue of whether to continue it is to some extent one of economics, as discussed above. The question to be considered is: How much should one be prepared to pay, to ensure that only $x\%$ of cases of SNHL remain undiagnosed after a specified age—and how does this sum relate to the overall investment in children's audiology services?

  (c) Where there is no formal or effective neonatal screen but a continued policy of distraction testing, purchasers should examine, or if necessary commission, an audit of how this procedure has performed over the past few years. We predict that any district which does not fulfil the conditions for high quality programmes set out on p. 154 will find, on detailed audit, that distraction testing has made little contribution to early diagnosis. The options in this situation are as follows:

(i) Make whatever investment is needed in staff, training, and information systems to raise quality, and review the results over the next 2 years.

(ii) When further relevant research findings are published, consider whether improvements to the distraction test (as discussed above) should be introduced on a trial basis.

(iii) Discontinue the distraction test. If this option is chosen, it will be important to consider what alternatives are available. Selective neonatal screening with improved parent information and easy access for all parents to an audiology clinic is one possibility. It must be accepted that such a programme will miss a small number of cases, but its performance may be comparable to that of the distraction test as currently carried out in many districts.

We emphasize again that setting up any neonatal screening programme is not easy. It should only be contemplated in districts where there is already a well-run audiology service, since considerable professional support will be required to initiate and run the screening programme and handle the follow-up consequences.

• **Impedance tests** should not be regarded as a screening procedure.

Research

Research is needed on many aspects of screening for hearing loss, including techniques, organization, and yield.

1. What is the most cost-effective approach to neonatal screening and to the detection of hearing loss not present at birth?
2. How certain are we that early intervention really improves outcome and what measures should be used to answer this question? Might there be any adverse effects of early intervention?
3. Does treatment improve the quality of life and behavioural outcomes of OME sufficiently to justify screening and, if so, which children would benefit most? Can we predict which children will suffer persistent OME?

Monitoring and outcomes

Single measures such as age of detection or age at fitting of first hearing aid in children with SNHL must be treated with caution for the following reasons:

- It can be difficult to define these points precisely.
- Ascertainment is often uncertain, particularly in areas of high population mobility. For example, 'missed' cases may eventually be detected in other parts of the country.
- Ascertainment is never complete until around 5 or even 6 years of age, even in districts with a good service; therefore mean ages of diagnosis or of aiding are always several years out of date and respond slowly to changes in service delivery.
- Dramatic improvements can be obtained in mean and median age of detection by introducing selective neonatal screening, and these figures may conceal other less satisfactory aspects of the detection programme. These figures can also be affected by the inclusion of a small but not insignificant number of babies who show evidence of hearing impairment during the neonatal period and are fitted with hearing aids but subsequently turn out to have normal hearing.

There is no substitute for comprehensive audit and quality monitoring of the performance of the audiological programme. It is important to keep under review not only ages of diagnosis, but false-positive referral rates, waiting times at each point in the network of services (including ENT), and the differences between age of diagnosis for high-risk and low-risk cases. Standardization of records would facilitate comparisons between districts.

Evaluation of screening programmes for hearing loss in childhood
It is difficult to evaluate the sensitivity of screening programmes for hearing loss because 'missed' cases may not be diagnosed for several years, by which time they may have moved to another district. The follow-up of very large cohorts of children to detect missed cases is difficult and prohibitively expensive. The creation of a national register of children with hearing impairment would (if well designed and adequately funded) help to overcome this problem in addition to providing other research opportunities.

Notes and references

A more extensive bibliography is available on hearing screening; see p. xi for details.

1. Davis, A. and Wood, S. (1992). The epidemiology of childhood hearing impairment: factors relevant to planning of services. *British Journal of Audiology* **26**, 77–90.

2. The following articles together provide an overview of screening and an extensive bibliography: Davis, A. (1995). Current thoughts on hearing screening. In *Recent advances in community paediatrics* (ed. N. Spencer). Churchill Livingstone, Edinburgh; Robertson, C., Aldridge, S., Jarman, F., Saunders, K., Poulakis, Z., and Oberklaid, F. (1995). Late diagnosis of congenital sensorineural hearing impairment: why are detection methods failing? *Archives of Disease in Childhood* **72**, 11–15; Davis, A.C., Wharrad, H.J., Sancho, J., and Marshall, D.H. (1991). Early detection of hearing impairment: what role is there for behavioural methods in the neonatal period? *Acta Otolaryngolica Supplement (Stockholm)*, **482**, 103–9.

3. The case against universal neonatal screening is argued by Bess, F.H., Wilkerson, B., and Paradise, J.L. (1994). Universal screening for infant hearing impairment: not simple, not risk-free, not necessarily beneficial and not presently justified. *Pediatrics* **93**, 330–4.

4. For a comprehensive review of middle-ear disease and its significance see Haggard, M. (1993). *Research in the development of effective services for hearing impaired people.* Nuffield Provincial Hospitals Trust, London; Haggard, M. and Hughes, E. (1991). *Screening children's hearing.* HMSO, London.

5. Fortnum, H.M. (1992). Hearing impairment after bacterial meningitis: a review. *Archives of Disease In Childhood* **67**, 1128–33.

6. National Deaf Children's Society (1994). *Quality standards in paediatric audiology*, Vol. 1, *Guidelines for the early identification of hearing impairment.* National Deaf Children's Society, London. (Describes the standard of service which should be provided.)

11

Screening for vision defects

This chapter:

- Describes defects likely to cause disabling impairment of vision
- Defines the terms used to describe the common disorders, such as squint, refractive error, and amblyopia
- Reviews the tests and procedures used for assessing vision in preschool children
- Sets out the arguments for and against screening
- Gives a brief account of colour vision defects and vision problems associated with 'dyslexia'
- Makes recommendations for screening and early detection

Disorders of vision can be subdivided into the following categories:

- serious defects likely to cause a disabling impairment of vision ranging from partial sight to complete blindness[1];
- the common and usually less incapacitating defects, including refractive errors, squints, amblyopia, and defects of colour discrimination.

Conditions causing a disabling vision impairment as the primary problem

These are individually and collectively uncommon, with a combined incidence of 2–5 cases per 10 000 births.[2] This figure underestimates the prevalence of visual impairment in the community because there is under-reporting of children who have cortical vision defects with multiple other impairments.

Early detection is important

Detection of serious visual impairment is important for four reasons:

1. Some conditions are treatable, for example retinopathy of prematurity, cataract, glaucoma, and retinoblastoma. This also applies to

some acquired eye disease, notably uveitis in association with juvenile chronic arthritis.

2. Many visual disorders have genetic implications.
3. Developmental guidance and early educational advice by specialist teachers is much appreciated by parents and probably reduces the incidence of secondary disabilities such as behaviour problems. Multidisciplinary support may be needed for children with additional impairments.[3]
4. Ophthalmic symptoms or signs such as squint or progressive visual failure are occasionally the presenting feature of serious systemic disease.

How early detection is achieved

Many cases are detected by parents or other family members. A significant number are found at the neonatal examination by simple inspection of the eyes. Some are found by specialist examination of known high-risk groups, including low birth-weight infants at risk of retinopathy of prematurity, and babies with a first-degree relative known to have a potentially heritable eye disorder.

Screening for common non-incapacitating vision defects

Definitions

The terms used in this section are defined in the box. The most important of these is amblyopia, and the prevention, identification, and referral of this condition should be the main aims of a preschool vision-screening programme.

Amblyopia

Untreated amblyopia results in permanent vision impairment. Although this is usually (although not invariably) in only one eye, it may be a bar to certain careers and may leave the individual effectively partially sighted if the other eye is lost through disease or trauma. It has been estimated that this happens to approximately 30 people per year in the UK.

Definitions of terms used in the text
Visual acuity is a measure of how well a person is able to separate adjacent visual stimuli. Techniques that rely on the infant's looking behaviour are used in specialist centres, but all readily available methods require the subject's cooperation. The standard by which all other measures of visual acuity are judged is the Snellen letter chart (but see p. 169).

A **refractive error** is a disturbance of the optical system of the eye, such that a sharp image is not formed precisely on the retina. There is a genetic element in the development of conditions such as hypermetropia (long sight). The direct measurement of refractive error involves the technique of retinoscopy, for which cycloplegic agents must be instilled in the eye to paralyse accommodation. Techniques for the automated and semi-automated detection of refractive error are under development, but these cannot currently be recommended for the universal screening of infants. Few eyes form a perfect optical system and most people have some refractive error, which may change considerably in infancy and continues to alter throughout life. There is no precise relationship between refraction and visual acuity, and the decision as to when a refractive error should be regarded as abnormal depends on clinical expertise and judgement.

Myopia (short sight) is uncommon in infancy but becomes more common in late childhood and the early teens. It stabilizes in the early twenties and thereafter there is little change. **Hypermetropia (long sight)** is physiological until the age of around 2. In **astigmatism** the degree of refractive error is different between the two axes of the eye. **Anisometropia** means that the degree of refractive error is significantly different between the two eyes.

The **correction of impaired visual acuity** related to refractive error usually involves the prescription of spectacles. Severely impaired visual acuity may affect school work and sporting prowess, but minor impairments caused by slight refractive errors seem to have little impact on education or performance. Children are often reluctant to wear spectacles prescribed for these minor errors.

A **manifest squint** is a squint which is apparent at the time of examination. It is demonstrated by use of the cover – uncover test. The prevalence of squint in infancy is around 1% and in early childhood is between 3% and 7%. Squint is important for two reasons: it predisposes to amblyopia and impaired binocular vision; the appearance of a squint is distressing and therefore correction for cosmetic reasons is justified.

A **latent squint** is one which is detected only when the two eyes are dissociated by testing, using the alternate cover test. It may become manifest under conditions of stress, fatigue, or illness.

> **Amblyopia** refers to a condition of poor vision in which the eye itself
> is healthy, but because of a refractive error, a difference in refraction
> between the two eyes, a squint, or opacities in the refractive media,
> the brain has either suppressed or failed to develop the ability to per-
> ceive a detailed image from that eye. It is usually unilateral but may
> be bilateral in some circumstances, e.g. meridional amblyopia due to
> unrecognized astigmatism.

Amblyopia may be suspected in infants who present with other eye
problems such as squint, but is difficult to diagnose with confidence in
the clinical situation before the child can cooperate with visual acuity
testing. Prompt referral of infants with squint or other obvious vision
problems may help to avoid the development of amblyopia or reduce
its severity. In many cases, however, amblyopia presents for the first
time after the age of 3 without any other obvious signs of eye problems.

Treatment
The management of amblyopia often involves correction of refractive
error and patching, but is not entirely satisfactory; although gains in
visual acuity may sometimes be achieved, they are not always maintained, nor can the development of binocular vision be guaranteed.[4]

Treatment is said to be more effective in younger children and to be
of doubtful benefit beyond the age of 7 or 8. However, some authorities question whether treatment is effective at all, postulating that
apparent improvements in vision are due to a combination of measurement artefact and perceptual learning rather than a true increase in
visual acuity. The question is clearly important, and a randomized trial
of treatment of amblyopia may be needed to settle the issue.

Prevention
The goal should be the **prevention** of amblyopia, by detection and
treatment in infancy of the more common antecedent causes, which
include refractive error and squint. Trials have been conducted using
retinoscopy or isotropic photorefraction to diagnose these defects in
the first year of life. These show that the provision of spectacles for
babies with hypermetropia reduces the incidence of squint and amblyopia[5]. However, the overall impact on the number of cases of these
conditions is small and further research is needed before such a programme could or should be introduced. Furthermore, refraction is
changing rapidly in infancy, and so close supervision and frequent

skilled monitoring would be needed for a successful early intervention programme.[5]

Criterion of success

At present, therefore, the immediate criterion by which the success of a preschool vision screening programme should be judged is its ability to *detect* amblyopia as early as possible rather than *prevent* it. The long-term aim is to reduce the number of children with permanent vision deficits; the achievement of this goal depends not only on screening but also on the effectiveness of, and compliance with, treatment.

Assessing vision in young children

The measurement of visual acuity in children under the age of 3 years

The need for cooperation makes this very difficult. The method of forced choice preferential looking is only suitable for specialist assessment. Various tests have been used to demonstrate that the child has reached a developmental stage at which visual fixation and concentration on tiny objects is possible. These provide a *qualitative indication* of visual function, but cannot offer any measurement of visual acuity or any direct or indirect indication of refractive error. Examples include Sheridan's graded balls and matching toys tests, and the use of tiny sweets, known as hundreds and thousands (1 mm diameter).

Orthoptic examination   An orthoptist can observe whether the eyes work together as a pair and can test the ability of each eye to take up fixation. Although no direct measurement of visual acuity can be made in infancy, inferences can be drawn about the likelihood of significantly impaired vision in either or both eyes. The orthoptic examination requires a high level of skill, and it is naive to imagine that other staff can learn these techniques without thorough training. However, the orthoptic examination of every infant during the first year of life has a very small yield and is not currently thought to be justified.

Conclusion   There is currently no satisfactory way of assessing visual acuity suitable for the universal screening of children too young to cooperate with acuity tests.

The preschool child: 3–5 years

Between the ages of 2 and 3 years, children become more able to co-operate with vision testing. Although it is usual to test distance vision at 6 m distance, testing at 3 m gives acceptable results. It is often easier to maintain rapport and attention control at the shorter distance when testing young children, and many clinic rooms are too small for testing at 6 m.

The visual acuity for distance vision can be assessed using picture tests (Kay, Elliott), single letters (the *Stycar test* or preferably the *Sheridan Gardiner cards*) or a *Snellen chart*. Any of these can be used with a letter-matching card or with plastic letters so that the child does not have to be able to name the letters. A Snellen chart is preferable to single letters because the latter may seriously underestimate amblyopia (the so-called 'crowding phenomenon') or even miss the diagnosis altogether. It is essential to occlude each eye in turn, otherwise the result indicates only the vision in the better eye.

The *Cambridge crowding cards and the Sonksen–Silver test of visual acuity* overcome many of the disadvantages of existing tests. Both tests measure much the same thing and are validated for 3 m rather than 6 m. The Cambridge crowding cards have the additional advantage that the child only has to concentrate on the central letter in the array.

The Snellen chart, although widely regarded as the gold standard for visual acuity testing, has several defects. The progression of letter sizes on the chart is irregular, the number of lines on the chart increases with each step so that the task becomes relatively easier with larger letters, and the scale is too coarse for precise measurement of small changes. These problems have been overcome by the use of the log-MAR charts. The *Glasgow acuity cards* were designed to combine the advantages of existing tests with those of the logMAR design. They have yet to be evaluated in detail.[6]

The routine testing of *near vision* adds very little to the detection of significant visual defects. Children with hypermetropia do not necessarily have a significant reduction of near visual acuity. Near-vision testing can safely be omitted from the vision screening of children, although it does of course have a place in the assessment of the child with a suspected visual problem.

Coverage and cooperation Although it is important to design the best possible test for children, the limiting factor with preschool screening is the difficulty in obtaining cooperation when testing the less mature or mildly delayed child, resulting in unacceptably high recall or false-positive rates. Around 80 per cent of children can cooperate with vision testing at 3 years of age, and the figure rises to 90 per cent by 3¼.

In practice, a greater difficulty is in maintaining high coverage rates, with few screening studies reporting rates above 60–75 per cent.

Referral criteria   If the child can only read letter size 6/12 or less on the Snellen chart in either eye, despite good co-operation, referral is advisable. The referral criterion is 6/9 when single letters are used, provided that cooperation is satisfactory. The child should be reviewed if the vision is unequal but the vision in the worse eye is better than 6/12.

Is there a case for preschool screening for vision defects?

Vision screening before age 3 is very difficult for the reasons outlined above. Thus 'preschool' in this context means from age 3 until school entry, which is now commonly before 5 years of age.

Although the disability caused by impaired visual acuity in early childhood is not known, the experience of older children and adults suggests that correction of a visual acuity of 6/12 or worse is likely to improve quality of life. The disability and economic loss caused by squint and amblyopia are difficult to measure, and therefore the benefits of diagnosis before the child goes to school cannot easily be assessed. Nevertheless, there are two other arguments in favour of preschool vision screening:

- treatment for amblyopia can be initiated and sometimes completed before the child starts school;
- the results of intervention might be better.

It is difficult to quantify the benefits from the first of these. A child might be reluctant to wear a patch at school, but this may not always be necessary.

The second is an important and difficult issue. If the treatment of amblyopia is more successful at 3 than 5, early diagnosis would be important. Evidence to date suggests that age of starting treatment for amblyopia makes little difference to outcome within this age range.[4] However, amblyopia diagnosed at 3 years is often associated with squint, whereas when diagnosed at 5 years it is more likely to be associated with straight-eyed anisometropia, so that the cases are not strictly comparable. Thus the question is not yet finally resolved.

School entrant screening

The detection of vision defects in school entrants is easier (and therefore cheaper) than in the preschool years for the following reasons:

- school children are a 'captive population' and high coverage can be achieved easily;
- children aged 4 and 5 can cooperate more easily than 3-year-olds with the vision test requirements.

Myopia is rare in preschool children but becomes increasingly common during the school years. In this age group, the standard Snellen chart can be used for most children; single letters may be needed for a few very anxious or developmentally immature children. The incidence of new cases of myopia and of other eye diseases or disorders in older children is relatively low and many children recognize for themselves that they may need spectacles. Therefore the value of vision screening in secondary schools is open to question. For further discussion see the Polnay Report (note 3, p. 107).

Detection of squints

The majority of manifest squints are first *recognized by parents or relatives*. The parents should always be asked whether they have noticed any squint, laziness, or turning of one eye. Some parents are incorrectly informed that squint is normal under the age of 6 months, and this can lead to delay in diagnosis of serious eye disease. A family history of high refractive error or squint in a first-degree relative may be significant and justify referral for more detailed examination. The detection of squint is summarized in the box.

Community screening—evidence and options

Universal screening by an orthoptist of all infants in the first year of life would result in detection of some vision defects that would otherwise be missed. The yield would be very small and would not justify this use of an orthoptist's expertise. *Universal screening of all preschool children by doctors or health visitors* has a significantly

---

Detection of squint

A **careful inspection** of the eyes should be made to identify any squint which has been overlooked or ignored by the child's parents.

Some squints are not instantly apparent to simple inspection. In order to demonstrate these, the following tests may be used:

- the corneal reflections test
- the cover – uncover test
- the prism test
- examination of the eye movements, by moving a small target of visual interest through the horizontal, vertical and oblique planes
- stereopsis tests (e.g. Frisby, Lang, random-dot)

Some or all of these procedures could be used for screening, but the skill required for their proper performance and interpretation is not generally appreciated.

Pseudosquint A common difficulty is the distinction between squint and pseudosquint (i.e. the appearance of squint caused by epicanthic folds). Squint and prominent epicanthic folds may coexist. Pseudosquint is a very common reason for referral to children's eye clinics.

Screening for **latent squint** involves the use of the **alternate cover test**. It is doubtful whether the detection of a latent squint before it becomes a problem clinically is of any significant benefit to the child.

---

lower yield, and less satisfactory sensitivity and specificity, than a programme involving orthoptists[7]. Therefore the latter could offer a more effective service. At present, however, *we do not think that universal screening could be recommended*, in the absence of any evidence that this produces a better outcome in terms of visual acuity.

A community-based orthoptist may undertake *secondary screening* by examining children referred by parents or by other professional staff and selecting those who require a more detailed assessment. In this sense, a community-based orthoptic service might be better regarded as *an outreach from the ophthalmology service* rather than as a true screening programme. It appears to be cost effective since it results in a substantial reduction in the number of referrals to ophthalmologists and considerable financial savings. It may also help to reduce inequity, as social class plays a significant part in determining age of referral for children with amblyopia.[4]

An *assessment of visual acuity at school entry* is routine in most districts. This is usually done by school nurses. The advantage of testing this age group is that near-universal coverage can be achieved for the first time since infancy.

Colour vision defects

Deficiencies in colour discrimination, primarily affecting the perception of reds and greens, occur in 8 per cent of boys and about 0.5 per cent of girls. Blue deficiencies and total colour blindness are extremely rare. The Ishihara test is widely used, although it is very sensitive and detects even very minor defects which might be of trivial significance. The City University test is preferred by some. Two reasons are advanced for the early detection of colour vision defects.

1. It has been suggested that they might cause learning difficulties, particularly with regard to colour-coded materials used in the teaching of reading and mathematics. There is in fact little evidence that colour vision defects cause learning difficulties, and most affected children can distinguish different coloured materials despite reduced colour discrimination.
2. Some defects preclude people from entering certain careers, and it is helpful for a person to know that they have this deficiency at an early stage in career planning.

Screening at the beginning of secondary schooling might be useful, by providing information that would be important in career planning. A case can be made for including only boys, in view of the much higher incidence.

Little is known about whether adolescents benefit from or value this screening process. It might be equally effective to provide health education. For example, those whose career planning might be affected by colour vision impairment could be advised to visit an optometrist for assessment. See the Polnay Report for further discussion.[7]

Vision and 'dyslexia'

There has been much interest in recent years in the relationship between visual deficits, such as eye-movement disorders and delay in establishment of dominance, and dyslexia or reading problems.[8] A disorder known as 'scotopic sensitivity syndrome' has also been described.

The evidence on these conditions is still equivocal and further research is needed. There is no dispute that any child with reading or other learning problems needs a vision assessment, but we do not think that this need include tests or treatment for the conditions mentioned above, except in the context of a special development or research programme.

Recommendations

Recommendations for detection of severe visual impairment

- **A careful inspection of the eyes is a mandatory part of the neonatal examination.** Fundoscopy is not essential but the ophthalmoscope may be used with a +3 lens from a distance of 8–12 inches, to detect cataract as a silhouette against the red reflex. The inspection and the examination should be repeated at 6–8 weeks. Urgent referral is mandatory if there is any suspicion of abnormality.
- **The parents should be asked if there is a family history of visual disorders.** Children at risk of having a genetically determined disabling visual disorder should be examined with extra care, preferably by an ophthalmologist.
- **Parents should be asked soon after the birth and at each subsequent contact whether they have any anxieties about the baby's vision.** An age-related check-list in the personal child health record can be used. For example, they can be asked if the baby looks at the parents, follows moving objects with the eyes, and fixates on small objects.
- **Primary health care team staff should be familiar with the visual development of the normal baby,** and should be alert to the various symptoms and signs which first warn parents that there may be a visual defect, for example abnormal appearance of the eyes, wandering eye movements, poor fixation and visual following, photophobia, etc.
- **Children with dysmorphic syndromes or neurodevelopmental problems should undergo a specialist eye examination as some may have serious defects of vision.**
- **Babies with a birth-weight of less than 1500 g, or born at 31 weeks gestational age or less, should be screened for retinopathy of prematurity** according to current recommendations. The increased risk of other eye problems, including myopia, squint, and cortical visual impairment, should also be remembered.

- It should be remembered that poor visual fixation in the first year of life is sometimes the presenting feature of learning disability (mental handicap) rather than of an eye disorder.

Screening for non-disabling visual defects[9]

- Screening for non-disabling visual defects in children under 2 years of age should be confined to history and observation.
- Children of any age with suspected vision defects, a significant family history, or any neurological or disabling condition should be referred routinely for visual assessment.
- A visual acuity test should be carried out at school entry.
- Any child undergoing assessment for educational under-achievement or other school problems should have a visual acuity check.
- It is important to ensure that vision screening is undertaken in schools for children with hearing impairment because (a) good vision is particularly vital for a person with impaired hearing and (b) conditions such as Usher's syndrome, which have important genetic and educational implications, may present with insidious loss of vision.[10]
- One person in each district should take responsibility for monitoring the results of vision screening.
- Community-based secondary screening or outreach services by an orthoptist in the preschool age group (3¼–5) are probably worthwhile and cost effective, but the value of vision screening by other staff is more limited.
- The benefits of primary screening of all preschool children are still uncertain and it is very difficult to achieve adequate population coverage.
- The relevance of more subtle eye problems to reading difficulties and 'dyslexia' is controversial. Screening programmes for such problems could not currently be justified, but ophthalmology and paediatric services must decide how to respond to parents who are worried about this possibility.

Colour vision defects

- No attempt should be made to screen for colour vision defects in primary school.
- The value and timing of screening for colour vision defects in older

children is uncertain, although between 9 and 11 years is the most usual choice.

- **Children found to have a colour vision defect should be told** that they have a difficulty in discriminating colours which *might* be important with regard to certain career choices. In cases where the defect may have important career implications, **expert advice** should be obtained from an optometrist, an ophthalmologist, a specialist colour vision clinic, or a careers adviser.

Research

- The degree of disability caused by impaired visual acuity and amblyopia in childhood and later life needs further evaluation.
- Research is continuing on the development and evaluation of vision in infancy, with the eventual aim of preventing amblyopia.
- It will be important to confirm existing evidence that delay in diagnosis and treatment of amblyopia between the ages of 3 and school entry at age 4 or 5 does not seriously affect the outcome.
- The effectiveness of treatments for amblyopia is still uncertain and a randomized trial may be needed. This should also clarify the question of whether there are significant measurement artefacts (due to poor test – retest reliability) in assessment of vision in infancy.
- More detailed review of the potential savings, and service benefits, of community orthoptic services is needed.
- Visual acuity testing often presents practical difficulties in schools and there is undoubtedly scope for the development of new approaches.
- Many children now start school well before the age of 5. Screening of school entrants by an orthoptist or optometrist in schools might be more cost effective than either community-based preschool screening or school entrant screening by school nurses.
- The value of testing all secondary school children for visual acuity defects at age 14 has been questioned. It is said that adolescents are unlikely to wear spectacles unless they themselves recognize a visual difficulty. The alternative approach might be self-referral, encouraged by the inclusion of eye care as a topic in health education curricula. The benefits of this approach need further evaluation.
- It is not known whether children value and make use of the discovery

of a colour vision defect. An alternative approach which needs evaluation is to include eye care and colour vision defects in a health education lesson. Children who felt that such defects might be relevant to their career plans would be invited to attend for a screening test.

The role of optometrists

This review has concentrated on the value of the various procedures used for vision screening but has also considered the roles and skills of doctors, health visitors, and orthoptists. However, many children, particularly in the older age groups, have their vision tested by optometrists. Their contribution is important, and the most effective and efficient ways of coordinating the work of community child health services and optometrists deserve further evaluation.

Notes and references

A more extensive bibliography is available on vision screening; see p. xi for details.

1. Fielder, A.R., Best, A.B., and Bax, M.C.O. (1993) *The management of visual impairment in childhood.* Clinics in Developmental Medicine, Vol. 128. Blackwell Scientific Publications, Oxford.
2. DHSS (1988). *Causes of blindness and partial sight among children aged under 16, newly registered as blind and partially sighted between 1985 and 1987.* Statistical Bulletin no. 3/9/88. HMSO, London.
3. Moller, M.A. (1993). Working with visually impaired children and their families. *Pediatric Clinics of North America* 40, 881–90.
   Youngson-Reilly, S., Tobin, M.J., and Fielder, A.R. (1994). Patterns of professional involvement with parents of visually impaired children. *Developmental Medicine and Child Neurology* 36, 449–58.
4. The following papers describe a study of the treatment of amblyopia: Hiscox, F., Strong, N., Thompson, J.R., Minshull, C., and Woodruff, G. (1992). Occlusion for amblyopia: a comprehensive survey of outcome. *Eye* 6, 300–304; Woodruff, G., Hiscox, F., Thompson, J.R., and Smith, L.K. (1994). Factors affecting the outcome of children treated for amblyopia. *Eye* 8, 627–31; Smith, L.K., Thompson, J.R., Woodruff, G., and Hiscox, F. (1994). Social deprivation and age at presentation in amblyopia. *Journal of Public Health Medicine* 16, 348–51.
5. Atkinson, J. (1993). Infant vision screening: Prediction and prevention of strabismus and amblyopia from refractive index screening in the Cambridge Photorefraction Program. In *Infant vision: basic and clinical research* (ed. K. Simons), Committee on Vision, National Research Council, pp. 335–48. Oxford University Press, New York.

6. McGraw, P.V. and Winn, B. (1995). Measurement of letter acuity in preschool children. *Ophthalmic and Physiological Optics* 15, S11–S17.
7. There are a number of papers comparing various approaches to preschool screening: e.g. Bolger, P.G., Stewart-Brown, S.L., Newcombe, E., and Starbuck, A. (1991). Vision screening in preschool children: comparison of orthoptists and clinical medical officers as primary screeners. *British Medical Journal* 303, 1291–4.
8. Bishop, D.V. (1989). Unfixed reference, monocular occlusion, and developmental dyslexia–a critique. *British Journal of Ophthalmology* 73, 209|15.
9. The recommendations in this chapter are in line with those of a specialist joint working party: Royal College of Ophthalmologists and the British Paediatric Association (1994) *Ophthalmic services for children.* Royal College of Ophthalmologists and the British Paediatric Association, London.
10. Murdoch, H. and Russell-Eggitt, I. (1990). Visual screening in a school for hearing-impaired children. *Child: Care, Health and Development* 16, 253–61.

12

Disorders of development and behaviour

This chapter:

- Sets out the aims of child development programmes and describes the conditions and problems to be addressed
- Discusses the importance of identifying, detecting, and caring for children with disabling conditions
- Considers the early identification of speech and language impairments and behavioural problems
- Examines the role of developmental screening and routine developmental assessment
- Emphasizes the vital importance of collaboration between health, social services, and education in the planning of early identification activities
- Suggests priorities for service providers

In Chapter 5 we considered the primary prevention of developmental and behavioural problems and the promotion of parenting skills. Here we review the detection and management of conditions likely to cause disability and in some cases permanent handicap, i.e. secondary and tertiary prevention.

Disability

Disability* in childhood is an important problem: 1.8 per cent of children attend special schools and increasing numbers of disabled children attend mainstream school with additional support. Emotional and psychosocial problems are very common in childhood, and there are close relationships between a child's physical state, developmental progress, and mental health.

The prevention, identification, and management of disability involves many other disciplines and agencies in addition to those professionals directly concerned with child health. Recommendations which acknowledge the perspectives of social services, education

* The terminology used to describe disability is summarized in Chapter 1 (p. 15).

authorities and voluntary agencies are more likely to benefit children and should lead to mutual trust and better collaboration.

The conditions

The impairments to be considered may involve motor, intellectual, language, or emotional development. A wide variety of underlying conditions may be responsible, and the resulting disability may be trivial or profound, transient or permanent. Therefore it is impossible to propose any single solution to the problems of detection and diagnosis, early intervention, or long-term management.

In view of the very wide range of conditions to be considered, it is useful to distinguish two groups of problems.

- 'Low-prevalence high-severity' conditions: this group includes conditions for which a pathological basis has been demonstrated or can be presumed. Examples include cerebral palsy, aphasia, and severe learning disabilities (mental handicap).
- 'High-prevalence low-severity' conditions: this group includes delayed speech and language acquisition, clumsiness, and minor psychological pathology. A pathological basis for the child's difficulties is rarely found. They are assumed to be due to a combination of genetic and environmental factors, although in some cases neurophysiological 'processing' disorders are postulated.

The distinction is made for convenience and it is not claimed that it has any rigorous scientific basis. Some children in the second group may be more disabled than some of those in the first. However, there are some differences between these two groups in the approach to prevention, detection, and management.[2]

Low-prevalence high-severity conditions

These conditions, although rare, have serious effects on the individual child and collectively present a significant health care challenge to society. Details of the most common are shown in Table 12.1.

Primary prevention

There is little scope for primary prevention of these conditions within child care services. Prevention of brain damage by screening for

Table 12.1 Conditions causing disability in childhood

- Cerebral palsy: 0.15%–0.3% (1.5–3 per 1000)
- Duchenne muscular dystrophy: 0.03% of males (3 per 10 000 male births)
- Severe learning disabilities (previously mental handicap): 0.37% (3.7 per 1000)
- Speech and language impairments, including developmental and acquired dysphasia, pseudobulbar palsy, and unknown causes: incidence depends on the definition, but for persisting severe cases it is at least 2 per 1000
- Classic autism: 0.03%–0.04% (3–4 cases per 10 000 births)[3] Autistic spectrum disorder: 1–2 per 1000 (the number of children with severe communication problems included under this heading has risen in recent years and there is an excess of cases among the children of first-generation immigrants)
- In addition, there are a number of inherited disorders which may lead to disability, such as osteogenesis imperfecta, and many causes of acquired disability, such as head injury and juvenile arthritis

phenylketonuria and hypothyroidism has obvious benefits. The early recognition of genetically determined conditions such as Duchenne muscular dystrophy may avoid the birth of a second affected child within the same family. Prevention of acquired brain injury involves reducing risks of head injury by prevention of accidents and child abuse, prevention and prompt treatment of infections of the central nervous system, etc. (Chapter 3).

Periconceptional and antenatal health surveillance and health promotion

The health of the fetus and the parents during pregnancy has long-term effects on morbidity and mortality. The Working Party has not attempted to review this subject, but this is not to deny its importance. Preparation for parenthood, access to genetic counselling, family spacing, measures to reduce identifiable risks (such as rubella vaccination and folic acid supplementation), and sensible advice on alcohol, smoking, diet, and safe eating may all play a part in improving pregnancy outcomes and therefore the health of the child. The mental health of the parents, and in particular of unsupported mothers, is equally important. Support for mothers who have previously had a low birth-weight infant has been shown to have beneficial effects on a number of outcome measures. These topics are all relevant to Health of the Nation targets.

Detection

Although routine developmental examinations are capable of detecting extreme deviations from normal development, most serious impairments are found by other means (Chapter 5). The contribution of routine developmental reviews is very small.

High-risk follow-up

The early recognition of many children with cerebral palsy is facilitated by a high-risk follow-up clinic for neonatal intensive care (NICU) graduates. Between 8 and 20 per cent of cases of cerebral palsy are related to neonatal encephalopathy, and a further substantial proportion are related to the problems of prematurity and low birth-weight.[4] Diagnosis of hearing and vision defects and of moderate and severe motor impairments can usually be achieved within the first year of life, although the more subtle cognitive and behavioural problems associated with very low birth-weight may not be easily identifiable until

---

Correction for prematurity[4]

- In 1947, Gesell and Amatruda recommended that full correction for prematurity should be made when assessing the development of preterm infants. This seemed logical and is the usual practice.

- Normative data for available developmental tests were obtained on populations of mainly full term or slightly pre-term infants. The relevance of these data to very preterm infants is uncertain.

- If full correction is made for prematurity in the very pre-term infant, some infants with unequivocal motor abnormalities will have developmental quotients within the normal range. In other words, if developmental assessment is considered as a 'screening test' for cerebral palsy, the sensitivity is greater if no correction is made; specificity is greater if full correction is made.

- In the first year of life, for infants with no identifiable neurological deficit, prediction of IQ at age 5 is slightly better if scores corrected for prematurity are used; thereafter, prediction is better if uncorrected age is used.

- From the primary care team's perspective, there are two practical points. First, interpretation of developmental assessment in very preterm infants is difficult and usually needs specialist help. Second, concerns about development in general and motor development in particular in these infants should not be dismissed as being due solely to prematurity.

school entry or even later. In infancy, adjusting for prematurity complicates the monitoring of development and the interpretation of mild delays or deficits (see box). Follow-up of children who have experienced insults to the nervous system, such as trauma or infection, should identify a further significant proportion who are or become disabled.

Listening to parents

Inappropriate reassurance of parents by professionals continues to be a common cause of delay in diagnosis of disabilities. Staff should be familiar with the normal milestones of development and their variability, and with the various presentations of severe learning disabilities, muscular dystrophy, autistic spectrum disorder, etc., and should remember that in a significant number of these children (including those with cerebral palsy) no high-risk factors can be identified.

'Evolutionary' diagnoses

The period of uncertainty while a diagnostic problem evolves often leads to delay in commencing a formal intervention programme for children with cerebral palsy or severe learning disability. There is no evidence that this delay has any adverse effect on functional outcome, but the early involvement of therapy and educational disciplines is perceived by parents as highly beneficial and supportive, and this is particularly true in situations where the diagnosis is uncertain.

Communication

Above all else, parents value the quality of communication between themselves and the professionals.[5] Badly handled news-breaking is still one of the most common concerns voiced by parents of disabled children. This issue is important not only in cases where the child has a serious disorder but also when the problem is perceived by the professional to be relatively minor; it may not be minor to the parents.

Management

A comprehensive multidisciplinary service, usually though not invariably based in a child development centre, is essential for the assessment and care of these children.[6] Parents and voluntary organizations have made it very clear that they expect a high standard of investigation, counselling, support, respite care, and interprofessional communication. The conditions described are rarely amenable to treatment in the medical sense, but much can be done to improve quality of life.

High-prevalence low-severity conditions

Some impairments give rise to much concern in early childhood and are likely to affect educational progress, but are not sufficiently severe to prevent the attainment of independence in adult life. Many of these tend to improve as the child matures and some resolve completely. The most important of these, delay in speech and language acquisition, will be considered in some detail, for the following reasons:

- The identification of these children is one of the most contentious issues in preventive child health care at the present time and has important implications for social services and education authorities.
- It has been more extensively researched and debated than any other aspect of child development.
- It is likely that the conclusions drawn from research on this topic will be relevant to the whole child health promotion programme.

Other examples of developmental impairments include mild global learning disabilities, clumsiness, minor or mild psychological problems, and specific learning disabilities (see p. 15 for definition) such as 'dyslexia'.

Delay in speech and language acquisition

Normal variation

There are wide variations among normal children in the rate of language acquisition[7] (Fig. 12.1). Similarly, there are differences in the way that children acquire language. Genetic influences play a substantial role in determining the rate of language development (p. 180) and, at least within the normal range, socio-economic factors seem less important. Very fast developers are more likely to be found in professional families and extremely slow developers are more likely to have parents who are poor and in unskilled or semi-skilled jobs, but these are generalizations and the relationship is much weaker than is generally believed.

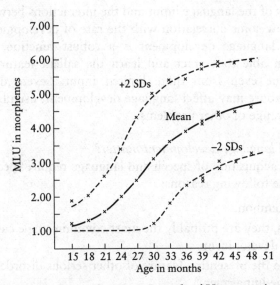

Fig. 12.1   The figure shows the Mean Length of Utterance (a standard measure of language production which is roughly equivalent to the number of syllables per sentence) plotted against age. The variability between children is such that one-sixth of children aged 4 years have an MLU equal to the 50th centile for a 3-year-old; in other words, one child in six can be said to be one year behind in expressive language development.

Reproduced with permission from Wells, G. (1985). *Language development in the preschool years.* Cambridge University Press.

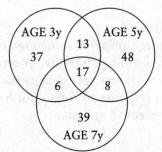

Fig. 12.1 (contd.)   The language development of 857 children was assessed at 3, 5, and 7 years. Many children were 'delayed' at one assessment, but only 17 were considered delayed at all three.

Reproduced with permission from Silva, P.A. (1987). *Epidemiology, longitudinal course, and some associated factors, an update.*

Clinics in Developmental Medicine, Vols 101/102, p.6. Blackwell Scientific Publications, Oxford. In *Language Development and Disorders* (ed. W. Yule and M. Rutter).

The *quality* of the language input and the interactions between parent and child show some correlation with the rate of development (p. 65); nevertheless, language development is a robust function, and most children seem able to extract and learn the salient features of their mother tongue even from quite limited input. Severe deprivation, neglect, and abuse may affect language development, usually in association with a range of other problems.

Does delayed language development matter?
Delays in the acquisition of speech and language require special consideration for the following reasons:

- They are common.
- For parents, they are probably the most common single cause of concern about development.
- They can be the presenting feature of other serious disorders (secondary language impairment).
- Severely impaired children may need special educational facilities.
- Intervention at an early stage might avoid irreversible impairment of language acquisition.
- Early developmental problems, psychosocial and behavioural problems, and environmental adversity may interact to create a series of negative experiences for the child and parents which seriously affect subsequent health and progress. Early intervention might break this downward spiral of disadvantage.

Secondary language impairment
In some children language delay is secondary to other impairments, such as deafness, severe learning disability, or cerebral palsy, and there are also a few children with very rare deficits such as auditory agnosia (children who show no response to sound but have normal peripheral hearing) and acquired receptive aphasia.

Co-morbidity
Delayed language development may be an isolated phenomenon, but it is commonly accompanied by other problems such as generalized cognitive impairment, behaviour and conduct disorders, and attention deficits. Cognitive deficits (low IQ) impose a limit on the rate of language development (with rare exceptions), but conduct and attentional problems are best regarded as associations or 'co-morbidity'.

Specific language impairment

Many authors have drawn a distinction between 'delayed language development' and 'language disorder', but there are no absolute differences between these categories[9] and the value of distinguishing them is doubtful. The term 'specific language impairment' (SLI) is preferred by many authorities. Operational definitions of this term vary between authors, but all acknowledge the fact that a child can have difficulties with one or more aspects of the use of language which are out of keeping, or out of step, with other intellectual functions and are not explained by hearing loss or overt neurological disorder. The causes of impaired language development, though widely debated, are still uncertain (Table 12.2).

Assessing outcomes for language-delayed children

The current interest in delayed language acquisition[10] results from studies in the 1970s and early 1980s, which showed that delayed onset of language is strongly associated with academic problems, reading difficulties, behavioural disorders, and continuing language deficits. Until recently, few research studies made the distinctions that are now recog-

Table 12.2 Correlates of language impairment (LI)

- Gender: LI is three to four times more common in males
- Genetic factors: play a part in persisting language delay—effects on transient expressive delay are less clear
- Laterality: probably not relevant
- Perinatal history: probably little or no relevance
- Motor deficits: suggested by association with drooling and choking, and with fine motor problems
- Middle-ear disease: may be important for individual children but not responsible for the majority of cases of LI
- Family size and birth order: large families may cause relative deprivation of verbal interaction with adults
- Socio-economic status: highly significant relationship between poverty/socio-economic status and LI
- Verbal interactions in family: complex relationship; child's delay may affect parent's language as well as the parent having an influence on the child; linguistic environment is rarely the only cause of LI; bilingualism in itself is not a cause of LI though in some social contexts it may contribute.
- Behaviour and discipline in the home: complex relationship; frustration and lack of comprehension play a part but do not cause LI.

nized as crucial both for prognostic accuracy and for understanding of the relationships involved.[11]

- They did not control for IQ, i.e. they failed to separate the effects of low intelligence from those specific to language delay.
- They failed to separate the varying types and presentations of delayed language acquisition and in particular did not distinguish between delay in speech production (expressive delay) and recep-tive–expressive delay.[12]
- They failed to consider the size of the gap between non-verbal, expressive, and receptive skills. Categories of deficit are only mean-ingful if there are appreciable differences between these measures.

When IQ is controlled, delay in speech and language acquisition has in general a better prognosis than the early studies indicated.

Key issues in secondary language impairment

Although 20 per cent of parents are concerned about their child's speech development and 70 per cent of the country's speech therapy budget is spent on children, there is still little reliable information on which to base service planning. The following issues must be resolved.

- How should 'delay' or SLI be defined?
- What is the long-term significance of delay and SLI?
- Is intervention for SLI effective, and, if so, for which children, in what form(s), at what ages, and for how long?[13]
- Even if it is effective, is it *cost-effective*, i.e. might there be more educational or social benefit from investing in other forms of early intervention?

The questions are intimately related, since the definition of what con-stitutes a problem for the child should logically be governed by the extent to which prognosis is affected by early speech and language problems and whether or not they are amenable to intervention.

Definition of delay and SLI

There are no specific linguistic markers which distinguish between those children who will eventually develop normal language and those who will have continuing problems. In defining diagnostic criteria, the *wide variation in normal language acquisition* must be considered (Fig. 12.1).

Definitions based on the number of words used at a particular age are attractive in their simplicity, but children rarely present for clinical evaluation at convenient fixed ages. It is perhaps more useful to determine the limits of 'normality' by using standard deviation scores (cf. growth, p. 116). Some speech and language therapists have defined 'delay' as being more than 1 or 1.5 SDs below the mean, but such definitions will include large numbers of children. In the absence of evidence to the contrary, it might be more logical to follow accepted practice in other fields and use the 2 SD level as a marker of possible abnormality. However, in clinical practice additional factors must inevitably be taken into account, for example family history, coincident hearing impairment, or extreme parental concern.

Markers of language development
Although vocabulary size and early grammar are not the only indices of language development, they are probably the most useful in very young children and are certainly the easiest for parents and professionals to use. However, the difficulties and their clinical implications are illustrated by two contrasting definitions of 'delay'. The criterion of saying fewer than eight words at age 27 months (at least 2 SDs below the mean) identifies a small number of children with severe delay—the probability of spontaneous improvement over the next year is much less than in children with between eight and 20 words in their spoken vocabulary. In contrast, the broader criterion of fewer than 30 words and no word combinations at 24 months (equivalent to just over 1 SD below the mean) identifies between 9 and 17 per cent of children, depending on the population being sampled.[14]

Significance of slow language acquisition
Although there is some continuity in communication ability between infancy and early childhood, the long-term significance of delay in speech and language development at the age of 2 is quite limited. Only in cases of severe delay is concern about the child's future progress really justified.

The majority of children with expressive delay improve spontaneously (i.e. without formal intervention) and will function within the normal range by 5 years of age. Isolated problems in sound production or articulation are readily recognized by parents and professionals and cause much anxiety, but have an excellent prognosis in the majority of cases. Expressive SLI in the preschool period is better characterized as a risk factor than as a disorder. There seems little justification for actively seeking and referring 2-year-olds whose expressive language is only 1 or 1.5 SDs below the mean.

Comprehension deficits
These are easily overlooked by parents because children are often good at responding to non-verbal or situational clues. Nevertheless they are important, firstly because there may be an unrecognized hearing loss and secondly because they are more likely to be associated with long-term problems.

Relationship of speech and language delay to reading problems
The link between language delay and reading problems described in earlier studies is partly accounted for by the fact that these studies included children with low IQ. Nevertheless there is some link between early delay in language development and later under-achievement in reading and language-based skills, although this is rarely of sufficient severity to be regarded as an educational problem in its own right. There is also a more specific connection between deficient 'phonologic awareness' (detected by difficulties with games involving rhyming words) and reading problems (p. 66).

Long-term prognosis
The long-term prognosis is variable. Language deficits may persist and may cause considerable difficulties even in secondary school, but often go unrecognized and may present as psychological or educational problems.

Autism, Asperger's syndrome and autistic spectrum disorder
Children with severe impairment of *all* communication skills present a much more worrying picture. They may have severe learning disabilities and/or may be part of the *autistic spectrum*. In addition to delay in language development, difficulties with gestural communication (particularly protodeclarative pointing, i.e. with intent to communicate), pretend play, and social behaviour are observed in such children. These problems are often not recognized by professionals and surprisingly often are accepted as normal by parents, at least until the child is well past the second birthday. Early recognition may be possible if primary health care staff are aware of these features.[15] It is not yet known

whether this would have any benefits in terms of better outcome for the child or family.

Identification

Parents often know little about normal language development. Even highly educated parents may benefit from guidance and information. There is a natural tendency to focus on the quantity and clarity of speech, and professionals need to appreciate and explain the importance of *comprehension and social communication*. This information should be made available in a form accessible to parents, particularly at around the age of 2 when most children are starting to make rapid progress in language acquisition. It is important to educate parents about *hearing behaviour* and the need to assess hearing in any child with language delay, particularly if comprehension is suspect (p. 159).

Formal screening is not needed to identify children whose speech and language development is obviously normal or those who, equally obviously, have gross delay or abnormal development. The child's difficulties may be highlighted by a health professional, playgroup or nursery leader, or a friend or relative. Parents may need guidance in defining the nature of the problem, although they are often aware that the child is 'different'. However, in some borderline cases it may be difficult to decide whether further assessment is needed.[16]

In these circumstances, it may be necessary to refer the child for more specialist assessment. A 'screening' instrument for speech and language delay might have a role in this situation. This could reduce the number of referrals, provide a means of monitoring progress, and give parents and primary health care professionals the confidence to defer a formal assessment by specialists. This is a desirable goal because an excessive emphasis on very early referral of children who are slow to talk results in services being overwhelmed, long waiting lists, and consequently high non-attendance rates.

The identification of children with comprehension deficits may be important, and this can be difficult even for experienced professionals without the aid of a formal checklist or test. Several new 'screening' tests and procedures have been introduced recently, but their place in child health promotion is yet to be established.[17]

The identification of speech and language problems presents a difficult challenge when the family's mother tongue is not English. Staff dealing with this situation need to be well informed about the significance of bilingual environment. Specialist services such as speech and language therapy must be capable of carrying out assessments of such children using either a bilingual therapist or an interpreter.

The impact of universal nursery education   This should help early identification of, and intervention for, children with problems likely to affect learning and school progress.[18] If the full benefits of early nursery education are to be realized, greater efforts by health and education professionals will be needed to involve parents in their children's early education. A leading North American writer noted that:

In the future, health professionals, mental health professionals and educators may be able to collaborate to provide continuity of care, education and support to young children in ways that will make screening obsolete. A longitudinal, developmentally oriented care and educational system could be far superior to any cross-sectional screening approach for meeting the needs of young children in general and children with special problems in particular.[19]

Intervention

Parents vary widely in how much they know and are concerned about language acquisition. Whatever the nature of their concern, it is important to take it seriously and provide helpful and accurate advice. In determining whether intervention for delayed speech and language development is worthwhile, it is important first to define the aims. In addition to alleviating parental anxiety, these might be as follows:

(1) to treat and 'cure' the underlying processing deficit which is presumed to exist;
(2) to teach the child those specific components of language which are currently lacking, thus making the child more proficient at that point in time, but without necessarily expecting any long-term benefit.
(3) to give the child strategies to circumvent his language difficulties.

The last of these may be useful for older children with the insight to use such methods, but for young children the focus is either the first or the second. The fact that some language deficits persist into the school years (even though they may be subtle), and probably into adult life, hints that the first aim is over-ambitious in the present state of knowledge. Therefore aim (2) is probably the most realistic.

There are several approaches to intervention for children with SLI:

• placement in nursery or school environment with varying levels of specialist language support either on an individual basis or in a small group of children with SLI;

- clinic-based speech and language therapy, usually on a one-to-one basis or working in small groups;
- home-based therapy using the parent as agent under the guidance of the speech and language therapist
- a home-visiting programme such as Portage, usually oriented more to overall cognitive development rather than specifically to language.

These can be used separately or in combination.

Evaluation of intervention   This presents great difficulties. In contrast with the immense range of descriptive and analytic work on child language development, there are relatively few published intervention studies and hardly any randomized trials. Professional reluctance to include a control group receiving minimal or no intervention has contributed to the continuing uncertainty about the value of early intervention, with corresponding doubts about how much effort should be devoted to early detection. The findings of published research are summarized in the box but much remains to be done and the research problems are formidable.

- The range of severity is wide.
- The rate of spontaneous improvement is variable.
- There are many differing profiles of language delay, each with a different prognosis.
- Controls for non-verbal IQ and socio-economic status are essential.
- Apparent short-term gains with intervention may 'wash out' over time so that longer follow-up may reveal a diminishing advantage for the intervention group against controls.
- Conversely, there may be 'sleeper' effects, i.e. there may be no apparent benefit in early childhood but the advantages of early intervention might be seen in the teens or adult life.
- Single case studies can contribute useful information but it must be shown that the findings generalize to other children.

Interventions for speech and language problems

- Specific speech and language teaching procedures can accelerate the child's acquisition of vocabulary, phonological skills, and grammatical structures, but there is little evidence that these changes confer any long-term benefit to the child. This may be because of continuing spontaneous improvements in many untreated children, but the necessary long-term studies have not been performed. Little is known about the length of treatment needed for maximum benefit or the extent to which treatment generalizes to other areas of language.

- There is no apparent correlation between the amount of therapy received in the preschool period and the occurrence or prevention of school problems for children with SLI.

- For children with expressive SLI there is a temporary advantage, but no measurable persisting benefit, from traditional clinic-based speech therapy starting at the age of 2.

- There is no evidence that children with SLI benefit either more or less from intervention than children whose language delay is secondary to other problems.

- Parents can carry out intervention programmes under the guidance of speech and language therapists; the results are probably as good as those obtained with one-to-one professional therapy, though not all parents are able or willing to do this.

- Most children are treated on the assumption that they will acquire language in the same way as 'normal' children. This may not be true for those with severe SLI, and different approaches may be needed, perhaps requiring a more individualized programme.

- Because of the association between language problems and other behavioural and attentional difficulties, intervention often needs a substantial behaviour management component.

- In cases of environmental deprivation, language delay may be the most visible of the child's deficits but rarely occurs in isolation. Effective intervention programmes should probably address the child's development and family situation rather than focusing solely on language.

- Verbal interaction between staff and children in a day nursery is often less than would be needed (in both quality and quantity) to bring about improvements. Day nursery placement should not be regarded as a 'treatment' for language delay of predominantly environmental origin, although it may have many other benefits for parent and child. More structured educational programmes are likely to be more beneficial.

- Communication groups in day nurseries may result in significant gains not only in communication skills but also in other aspects of cognitive development, attention control, and behaviour.

- SLI is not the only form of communication problem which may need intervention. Other examples include early recognition and treatment of speech impairments associated with cleft palate, palatal dysfunction and hypo- and hypernasality, and explanation and counselling for parents of preschool children with problems of fluency as this may reduce the incidence of true stammering in adult life.

Borderline or mild learning disabilities ('developmental delay')

Causes

This may be due to specific conditions, non-specific genetic factors, environmental 'deprivation', or, most commonly, to an association and interaction of such influences. In cases where biological rather than environmental factors are the basis for the child's problems, early intervention will be requested and expected by parents. Programmes such as Portage appear to have little effect on the overall pace of learning or the eventual IQ, but are a great help to parents in understanding and meeting their child's needs.

Deprivation in the social and physical environment is an important cause of retardation in the mild to moderate range and, at least in theory, is amenable to intervention.

Motor delay and 'clumsiness'

Delay in walking is most commonly a normal variant, and is often associated with bottom shuffling. The majority of late walkers who have neurological reasons for the delay have been identified before 18 months of age, although 50 per cent of boys with Duchenne dystrophy walk later than 18 months.

'Clumsiness' is the colloquial term used to describe children who have poor coordination, sometimes but not always associated with other developmental difficulties. The term 'dyspraxia' has recently become fashionable, but the preferred description (DSM-IV,R) is 'developmental coordination disorder'. The more obvious motor difficulties tend to resolve over time but subtle problems persist in many children and are accompanied by a variety of social and relationship difficulties in school. Various treatment regimes have been described, although the value of these in the longer term remains uncertain and the availability of the necessary expertise is limited.

Specific learning disabilities

Specific learning disabilities (see p. 15 for definition) are only rarely recognized in the preschool years, but are occasionally suspected when alert parents or nursery teachers recognize potential difficulties; this may be more likely to happen when there is a positive family history of disorders such as reading problems ('dyslexia'). Although there are links between delayed language development and reading problems (p. 66), these are not sufficiently well understood to be used for screening in routine clinical practice.[20] Schemes for the general promotion of reading skills and the early identification of reading problems in school look more promising.

Mild and minor psychological and behavioural problems

The terms 'mild' and 'minor' are comparative.* The problems described are clinically significant and represent a health care need. They include behaviours or distressed emotions which are common or normal in children at some stage of development. They become abnormal by virtue of their frequency or severity, or their inappropriateness for a particular child's age compared with the majority of ordinary children. Therefore they are more than the annoying behaviour displayed by most children at some time.

Characteristics of minor psychological problems

- They are clinically significant because they are a source of considerable misery and distress to the child and/or the parents. Although often described as 'mild' or 'minor', they reflect a poor quality of existence for many children and parents.
- They are relatively persistent. It is commonly assumed that children will grow out of such problems (presumably because they are similar in form to ordinary difficult behaviour which is often transitory), yet they are remarkably persistent over years. In young children some of these problems can develop into or predispose to psychiatric disorder later in childhood. However, to some extent, they may be susceptible to prevention and treatment.
- They tend to be polymorphous. They present with varying combinations of difficult behaviour, angry outbursts, restlessness, moodiness, irritability or nervousness, eating and sleeping difficulties, poor relations with other children, aggressive behaviour, unusual fads or habits, continence problems, and social sensitivities.
- There are also more discrete patterns or problems existing as single entities: enuresis, encopresis, feeding disorder of infancy or child-

* Some of this material has been used previously in D. Hall and P. Hill, Community child health services. In *Health care needs assessment* (ed. A. Stevens and J. Raftery), pp. 451–554. Radcliffe Medical Press, Oxford (1994). Acknowledgements to Professor Peter Hill.

hood, pica, sleep disorders, conduct and oppositional disorders within the family, separation anxiety, sibling rivalry, and transient tics.

• Psychological problems interact with physical ill health, and in many cases the distinction between organic illness and psychological disorder is far from clear.

These problems are common
About 20 per cent of children have significant psychological problems, of whom perhaps a quarter need psychiatric specialist assessment. The remaining 15 per cent have emotional, behavioural, or psychological abnormalities which are clinically significant, and may benefit from health care, but are not sufficiently severe to be regarded as psychiatric disorders (Table 12.3).

Rates are higher in inner cities, socially deprived families, boys rather than girls, children with learning difficulties, young children with delayed language development, children with other problems of health or development, and in adolescence rather than earlier childhood. Associated family relationship problems are common although not universal. They include marital discord/altercations/divorce, mental health problems in other family members, and parental coldness or irritability toward the child.

Persistence
Minor psychological problems are relatively persistent, particularly when linked with continuing abnormalities in family relationships. This is true even for young children. Nearly half the psychiatric disorders in 14–15-year-olds represent conditions which have persisted since childhood.

Table 12.3 Rates for particular problems in preschool children

---

• Waking and crying at night: 15%
• Overactivity: 13%
• Difficulty settling at night: 12%
• Refusing food: 12%
• For polymorphous preschool behavioural problems involving a combination of high activity levels, disobedience, tantrums, and aggressive outbursts, associated with tearfulness and clinging, a point prevalence figure of about 10% can be estimated among 3-year-olds

---

Identification
There are several short behavioural checklists which could be completed by parents. The Behaviour Checklist designed by Richman and the Behaviour Screening Questionnaire are perhaps the best known. The psychometric properties (p. 202) of these have been established. Nevertheless, there are serious doubts about the wisdom of embarking on a formal behaviour screening exercise. The problems which would be encountered are the same as those described for developmental screening (p. 201). In the present state of knowledge it is more sensible for advice to be offered when parents seek help or when a professional identifies serious difficulties in child rearing and has concerns about the parent's ability to cope with the child's behaviour.

Intervention
The key issues in deciding whether treatment is necessary are the child's age, the number of psychological (emotional, behavioural, or developmental) abnormalities present, and the severity of their expression.[21]

A single psychological abnormality does not necessarily indicate psychiatric disorder, although it can do in a minority of instances. Like indigestion or headache, a psychological abnormality can be a problem in its own right in some children but a symptom of underlying disease in others. The prognosis for untreated single problems is considerably better than for polymorphous problems. This distinction is important in planning treatment. An isolated problem can often be handled by a direct approach to the presenting problem. A polymorphous picture will need a more time-consuming approach which takes parental mental health or family relationships into account and may exceed the capabilities of many primary care teams.

The inverse care law again   The families who might benefit the most from help with psychological problems in their children are often unable to make use of the strategies suggested because of various constraints such as the following:

• The association with poor family relationships and poor parental mental health: this directly impairs the quality of parenting required to contain difficult behaviour and anxious insecurity in young children, and discourages discussion of emotional difficulties in older children and teenagers.

• Associations with social deprivation and poverty: for instance cramped housing conditions and shared bedrooms reduce the success rate of mainstream treatments applied to sleep problems, enuresis, or defiant behaviour.

Intervention is effective in some circumstances There is evidence for the effectiveness of specific interventions in enuresis, faecal soiling, oppositional, defiant, or antisocial behaviour, and sleep settling/waking difficulties.

How to provide the services needed

The potential volume of referrals for minor psychological problems could quickly overwhelm the specialist child psychiatry and psychology services. Therefore the effective use of available services is particularly important.[22] Primary care staff need to be aware of normal development and the variations that commonly occur, the conditions and factors which must be considered when deciding on the most appropriate referral, and the availability of expertise within the district.

Health visitors with appropriate training can work effectively with cooperative families where the child presents with the common isolated problems listed above. Difficulties with sleeping, eating, temper tantrums, toileting, enuresis and encopresis, and separation anxiety are the topics most frequently cited in reports of successful interventions by health visitors.

Services are generally inadequate for children whose problems do not respond quickly to simple intervention, or who have multiple difficulties yet are not considered to require formal psychiatric help. Several service models have been proposed, but it is not yet clear which, if any, of these would be effective. Possibilities include community-based teams (involving for example a paediatrician, psychologist, and nurse), outreach child psychiatry programmes, community psychiatric nurses and school nurses, or health visitors with special training in behavioural management. Some services deal with a range of conditions, whereas others offer help for specific problems such as sleep disturbances or enuresis. Whichever model is adopted, close liaison with colleagues in education and social services is essential.

Problems with applying the concept of screening to development and behaviour

The first Working Party identified a number of fundamental difficulties in applying the Wilson and Jungner criteria for screening programmes

200 Health for all Children

1. **The difficulty of defining who should be regarded as a 'patient' or 'case'** It is not possible to give precise incidence or prevalence figures for these conditions because they cannot be defined exactly. There is no absolute distinction between, for example, normal and abnormal speech, or between excessive clumsiness and acceptable motor competence; nor is there any precise age at which failure to achieve a certain milestone can be said to be abnormal. Whatever cut-off point may be selected for screening purposes, many normal children will 'fail' the test while some with significant problems will 'pass'. In practice, the decision to refer a child for more detailed evaluation depends not only on the objective results of the clinical procedure or test, but on two other factors.

- **The parents' views**—whether the parents themselves consider the child to have a problem affecting development. It is essential to understand and respect the way in which parents perceive their child and any difficulties in development before constructive discussion and planning can take place. Their perceptions are dependent, at least in part, on their educational background, social status, and expectations for their children.

- **Referral for learning problems** in school-age children is governed more by the *availability of and access to diagnostic and remedial services* than by any other factor, and this is probably also true of preschool preventive health care.

2. **The unpredictable natural history of developmental impairments in early childhood** Children do not all develop at the same rate, nor do they all follow the same sequence of development. They may show substantial discrepancies in the rate of progress in various aspects of development. For example, some of the children who walk late (i.e. later than 18 months) have a neurological disorder or a learning disability, but the majority will turn out to be normal. Conversely, children with significant abnormalities such as congenital spastic hemiplegia may achieve their developmental milestones well within the so-called normal range.

3. **The lack of evidence regarding the extent to which early intervention is effective** in changing the natural history of developmental problems. We could find no clear-cut criteria for identifying those children who might benefit most from early assessment and intervention.

4. **Inadequate facilities for assessment and intervention** Parents complain of long delays and shortages of therapy and remedial teaching, for example, in both the NHS and the education services.

to 'developmental screening'. These are listed in the Box. Many of these problems have already been illustrated in the section on Speech and language problems. Similar arguments apply to screening for other developmental and behavioural impairments.

Developmental screening tests

There are at least a dozen developmental screening tests in widespread use, and many more that are used in restricted areas. Psychometric and screening performance data (page 202) are available for only a few of these tests. The *Denver Developmental Screening Test (DDST)* (see box) is the best known.[23] Other methods have been used in the UK. Some professionals prefer not to use standardized tests at all. Others use a range of tests of which the *Schedule of Growing Skills* is perhaps the most popular.

The Denver test

The *Denver Developmental Screening Test (DDST)*, devised and recently revised by Frankenburg, is the most popular developmental screening test in North America and the best researched anywhere in the world. Extensive data are available regarding its psychometric characteristics and its performance as a screening test. The main failing of the first version of the test was its low sensitivity, i.e. it failed to identify a substantial proportion of the children who have significant developmental problems, it performed particularly poorly in the detection of language difficulties, and it was not effective in determining which children are likely to have educational difficulties (although this was a task for which it was not designed). The new edition, published recently, is a considerable improvement, particularly with respect to the content of language items. Nevertheless, the limitations of developmental screening instruments and the need for a wider approach have been reviewed recently by Frankenburg.

The DDST does not fulfil the rigorous requirements for a screening test which were set out on p. 83. There is no reason to suppose that other less well researched tests are superior.[24] Perhaps new tests could be designed with higher *concurrent* validity (see box); however, it seems unlikely that substantially superior *predictive* validity can be achieved because there are limitations to the predictive validity of even a complete psychological assessment in the first few years of life.

Developmental screening questionnaires which are completed by parents have also been investigated, since they have obvious attractions of convenience and economy. The results of some studies are promising, but it is uncertain how effective questionnaires would be for poor or uneducated families. Such questionnaires are an alternative method *of* screening, *not* an alternative *to* screening.

Definitions

Developmental examination—a clinical procedure which evaluates the level of development reached by a child at a particular age and detects any significant deviations from the normal. It may include an interview with parents, structured observations, physical and neurological examination, and the administration of specific tasks. Interpretation of a developmental examination relies on a comparison of the abilities of the child being examined with those of other children of the same age. The data about normal development which are needed to make this comparison are available in various developmental tests, charts, and scales.

Developmental screening—the performance of one or more developmental examinations on apparently normal children at specified key ages in infancy and early childhood. As with other screening tests, the aim is to examine *all* apparently normal children in order to identify those who may have some undetected abnormality. The term 'developmental screening' is restricted by some commentators to test procedures which are designed to meet the classic criteria for screening tests (p. 83). Thus, they should be simple to administer, so that they can be used by paramedical staff, they should have standardized test items, and they should include clearly defined pass–fail rules for referral. However, others have used the term to describe more extensive and sophisticated examinations which clearly do not meet the criteria for screening tests and are better described as assessments.

Assessment involves the detailed, expert, and often multidisciplinary investigation of manifest or suspected developmental delay or abnormality. In this situation, assessment is a diagnostic and problem-solving exercise. In educational terms assessment means the process of monitoring a child's level of performance, together with strengths and weaknesses, in order to establish an appropriate programme of teaching and to predict likely educational needs in the future. Defined in this way, assessment is not a problem-solving activity but an intrinsic part of good educational practice.

Psychometrics—the science of measuring human development, intellect and behaviour. In psychometric terms, a *test* is any systematic means of gathering and recording data about an individual. Therefore a structured questionnaire can fulfil the definition of a test. *Normative data* provide information about how other individuals perform in the test under consideration. *Reliability and repeatability* are measures of the extent to which the same results would be obtained by different testers, or by the same tester on different occasions. *Concurrent validity* is a measure of how much the test measures what it purports to measure. *Predictive validity* is a measure of how well the test correlates with certain specified outcomes.

Assessing the home environment

Assessment of the opportunities for play and learning available in the child's home might be useful when considering the need for support and professional intervention. Various methods have been devised for this purpose, but they have been used mainly for research and with a few exceptions have not become popular in clinical practice.

Assessment or screening?

Development is too complex a process to be measured by screening tests. An alternative approach is to provide for all children a series of detailed 'assessments' by a professional competent to carry out and interpret psychometric tests, make decisions about intervention, and offer counselling on health and child management issues. This approach could be justified only if it improved outcomes, for example more rapid school progress or a reduction in behaviour problems or exclusions from school.

Routine developmental assessments for all school entrants?

Development of policies for preschool surveillance and health promotion should be considered in conjunction with school health issues. When a child starts school, there are opportunities to identify any health or other problems that have been overlooked previously; furthermore, information on such findings can be used to monitor preschool services and identify any shortcomings.

It has been suggested that a neurodevelopmental examination at school entry may provide an effective vehicle for demonstrating a child's developmental difficulties and educational needs to both parents and teacher at school entry. We have not discussed this in detail since this and related school health issues have recently been reviewed in the Polnay Report (note 3, p. 107); however, we agree that detailed developmental assessment of all school entrants is unlikely to be justifiable in terms of yield or cost effectiveness.

Other methods are needed to ensure the early recognition of children who may need additional support in school. The teacher can use a checklist as a basis for reviewing each pupil. Suitable instruments exist and appear to be at least as effective as assessment by a health professional in ascertaining potential problems. This is to be expected, since they make use of the teacher's continuous classroom observation rather than being dependent on a single period of assessment.

This is an important area of research in education at present, because of the need to assess 'value added' (the educational equivalent of 'health gain') when comparing the performance of schools. Teachers need to know the abilities of their pupils when they start school, so that they can assess the amount of progress made when standard testing is carried out at the age of 7.

Measuring the effectiveness of routine developmental screening and assessment

We argued at the start of this report that child health programmes are too complex to evaluate as an entity; it is more profitable to consider each of the individual activities and tests separately. Nevertheless, there are some studies which set out to examine the overall effectiveness of child health programmes in a variety of ways (see pp. 71–3).

Identification of a problem, however precise, is not necessarily helpful; the ability to predict adverse outcome does not mean that the outcome will be improved. Even though preschool children with problems can be, and often are, correctly identified, this does not seem to improve their progress or behaviour measurably when assessed several years later. Possible reasons for the difficulty in demonstrating the value of developmental screening programmes are summarized in the Box. They do not constitute a reason for abandoning efforts to improve developmental and educational outcomes for children, but they do highlight the need for caution, the sensible use of resources, and cross-disciplinary collaboration in both service work and research.

A pragmatic approach—reconciling varying views by setting agreed priorities

We have tried to reconcile the research evidence, the understandable scepticism of purchasers and fundholders, the passionately held views of many professionals, the clearly expressed concerns of parents and voluntary organizations, and the duties laid upon statutory authorities by legislation. We suggest that there are three areas which should be

Possible reasons for difficulty in demonstrating benefit from developmental screening programmes

1. Are developmental conditions of trivial importance? Speech and language problems, developmental coordination disorder, reading difficulties, and some emotional and psychological conditions have significant implications for future development and mental health. However, if the criteria for 'a case' include children with minor or self-limiting difficulties, the possible benefits of intervention for children with more serious problems may be obscured.

2. Are the tests and procedures used inadequately designed or incorrectly administered? This may be true in part; there is room for improvement in the tests and a wide range of skill and commitment is found in their administration and interpretation.

3. Are the conditions detected by professional programmes equally well detected by other means? Although developmental examinations may result in conditions being detected before they are obvious to parents or others in contact with the child, any delay might be insufficient to alter the outcome.

4. Does the problem lie in the intervention offered rather than the detection process? Perhaps intervention is fundamentally ineffective or is provided 'too little and too late'; the available resources may be spread too thinly or not targeted to the children who could benefit the most.

5. Are the wrong outcome measurements being used? In other words, the satisfaction of parents and the support they receive from the programme could be the important benefits rather than changes in the child's development or progress.

6. Is the design of the published research projects insufficiently sensitive to detect important benefits? The greatest benefits of preventive programmes might accrue to families of the lowest socioeconomic status who are probably seriously under-represented in many research samples.

7. Do preventive health care programmes fail to reach the children who could benefit the most? The coverage of child health programmes is high in the first year of life, but thereafter falls progressively. Typically between 50 and 70 per cent of children in the 3–5 year age group participate in some form of preventive child health programme. The inverse care law applies: children who do not attend constitute a group at higher risk of problems and abnormalities.

8. Are the effects of social conditions and poverty so overwhelming that they swamp any benefit resulting from preventive child health programmes? There is no doubt about the importance of these factors as determinants of health, but we believe that this view is unjustifiably nihilistic.

regarded as priorities for service provision and that these should be seen to be done well before other tasks are attempted.

- *Identifying and helping children with permanently disabling conditions (listed previously) and providing support for their families* This can be accomplished by:
  - neonatal and 8-week examinations;
  - specialist follow-up of high risk babies;
  - responding promptly and sensitively to the concerns of parents, relatives, and other professionals (opportunistically or at routine child health surveillance reviews as set out in the core programme.

Many of these children will be identified within the first 2 years of life. Health professionals play an important role in early identification, but a coherent 'seamless' service, which parents demand, depends on the cooperation of health care providers, purchasers, and fundholders with the education authority and the social services department. Close collaboration is essential if the responsibilities placed upon these bodies by the Education Acts and the Children Act are to be properly discharged. There is more than adequate information about the type and standard of service wanted by parents, but wide variations still exist between districts.

- *The identification of children whose emotional, cognitive,and language development is being affected adversely by their environmental circumstances* Knowledge of which families are likely to be in this situation is vital in order to achieve this aim (see pp. 68–9). In this situation, appraisal of the parents' coping ability and the level of 'stimulation' in the home is essential. There is scope here for primary prevention as well as early intervention (see Chapters 2, 3 and 4 for more detailed discussion). Provided that adequate services are available, the prognosis for such children can be significantly improved.

- *The identification of children with developmental impairments which are known to have adverse prognostic significance* This category includes global learning disability (developmental 'delay'), generalized communication disorders (autistic spectrum disorder), and severe specific language impairment affecting both comprehension and expression, particularly when associated with behavioural and attentional deficits. The differential diagnosis includes hearing impairment, and all these children will need a hearing assessment. Children with these problems usually come to professional attention between 18 and 42 months of age. They are likely to need additional educational support, and it is helpful if they are identified and referred for educational assessment by the age of 3½. However, there is no value in identifying these children unless there is a well-organized service to receive referrals and provide appropriate educational and therapeutic intervention for them.

- *We would assign a lower priority to the use of developmental screening tests for all children and to the identification and referral of children with isolated mild or moderate expressive language delay* Although it would be surprising if this activity had no benefits at all, current evidence suggests that long-term outcomes do not justify the necessary investment of professional time.

Recommendations

- **The quality of the services provided for the assessment and management of children** with serious and disabling conditions should be reviewed and upgraded if necessary; effective medical and therapeutic care must be available; support, liaison with other agencies, fulfilment of statutory obligations, and links with voluntary organizations are also important.
- Since many conditions can be detected through **follow-up of high risk children**, arrangements should be reviewed to ensure that this happens and that children with serious disabilities are referred promptly for assessment.
- **Parents' worries** must always be taken seriously.
- Since **'news-breaking'** is perceived by parents as one of their greatest concerns and causes of distress, there is scope for tertiary prevention by improving the quality of professional–parent communication by appropriate training.
- Key professional staff, in particular health visitors, need **an extensive knowledge of normal child development and this must be updated regularly**.
- Although many of the children whose language development causes concern to parents and professionals will turn out to be normal, detection of those who do have significant problems is important and **prompt access to audiological services** and to **a speech and language therapist** is essential.

- **Parents should be provided with information,** together with support and help when needed, to understand normal development and language acquisition. Primary prevention of mental health problems is an important objective. It should be incorporated in service planning and regarded as a research priority.

- Primary care teams, and in particular health visitors, should be familiar with the various forms of **minor psychological problems** outlined above and should know how to assess the likelihood of a successful outcome with simple interventions.

- Whatever service model for mental health problems is chosen, we emphasize that there is little value in developing the skills of primary care staff **unless they can call on the help of a psychologist or psychiatrist** when faced with clinical problems outside their range of expertise.

- Programmes designed to help children whose development is causing concern, whether for 'biological' or social reasons, should not be solo efforts of the health services but rather a **combined initiative** involving health, education, and social services together with the voluntary sector.

- There is an urgent need to establish **multi-agency working groups** where these do not already exist.

- **Routine formal screening** for developmental problems, language impairment, or behavioural and emotional disorders is **not** recommended.

- There may be a role for a formal language screening instrument to be used on a selective basis, but at present this should be in the context of a carefully designed trial.[16]

- Children who are slow in language development may benefit from (a) **support, advice, and training for parents,** and (b) **communication groups** in nurseries and schools. These approaches may be at least as good as individual one-to-one therapy.

- Children with very severe difficulties in language development (whether SLI or secondary) may need a **different approach** in terms of both service delivery and the structure of the therapy and teaching programme.

Notes and references

A more extensive bibliography is available on speech and language disorders and development screening; see p. xi for details.

1. Two essential books on early intervention: Meisels, S.J. and Shonkoff, J.P. (1990). *Handbook of early childhood intervention.* Cambridge University Press; Guralnick, M.J., and Bennett, F.C. (ed) (1987). *The effectiveness of early intervention for at-risk and handicapped children.* Academic Press, Orlando, FL.
2. General reviews of developmental screening and surveillance: Bain, J. (1989). Developmental screening for pre-school children: is it worthwhile? *Journal of the Royal College of General Practitioners* **39**, 133–135; Colver, A.F. (1990). Health surveillance of preschool children: four years' experience. *British Medical Journal* **300**, 1246–8; Dearlove, J. and Kearney, D. (1990). How good is general practice developmental screening? *British Medical Journal* **300**, 1177–80; Dworkin, P.H. (1989). British and American recommendations for developmental monitoring: the role of surveillance; *Pediatrics* **84**, 1000–10; Frankenburg, W.K., Chen, J.H., and Thornton, S.M. (1988). Common pitfalls in the evaluation of developmental screening tests. *Journal of Pediatrics* **113** 1110–13; Meisels, S.J. (1988). Developmental screening in early childhood: the interaction of research and social policy. *Annual Review of Public Health* **9**, 527–50. Wearmouth, E.M., Lambert, P., and Morland, R. (1994). Quality assurance in preschool surveillance. *Archives of Disease in Childhood* **70**, 505–11.
3. Overview of autism: Gillberg, C. (1990). Autism and pervasive developmental disorders. *Journal of Child Psychology and Psychiatry* **31**, 99–120; Wing, L. (1988). The continuum of autistic characteristics. In *Diagnosis and assessment in autism* (ed. E. Schopler and G. B. Mesibov), pp. 91–110. Plenum Press, New York and London.
4. Pharaoh, P.O., Stevenson, C.J., Cooke, R.W., and Stevenson, R.C. (1994). Clinical and subclinical deficits at 8 years in a geographically defined cohort of low birthweight infants. *Archives of Disease in Childhood* **70**, 264–70. For references on correction for prematurity, see extended bibliography, p. xi for details.
5. Useful reviews on professional–parent communication: Sloper, P. and Turner, S. (1993). Determinants of parental satisfaction with disclosure of disability. *Developmental Medicine and Child Neurology* **35**, 816–25; Beresford, B.A. (1994). Resources and strategies: how parents cope with the care of a disabled child. *Journal of Child Psychology and Psychiatry* **35**, 171–210.
6. Robards, M.F. (1993). *Running a team for disabled children and their families.* Clinics in Developmental Medicine, Vol. 130. Blackwell Scientific Publications, Oxford.
7. Bates, E., Dale, P.S. and Thal, D. (1993). Individual differences and their

implications for theories of language development. In *Handbook of child language* (ed. P. Fletcher and B. MacWhinney). Blackwell, Oxford.

8. The effects of abuse on communication skills are complex. Neglect probably has the greatest impact on language development. See Law J. and Conway J. (1991). *Child abuse and neglect: a review of the literature.* AFASIC, London. (Available from AFASIC, 347, Central Markets, Smithfield, London EC1A 9NH, tel. 0181 236 3632/6487.)

9. Bishop, D.V.M. (1994). Is specific language impairment a valid diagnostic category? Genetic and psycholinguistic evidence. *Philosophical Transactions of the Royal Society of London B* 346, 105–11.

10. Useful books on language development: Fletcher, P. and Hall, D.M.B. (1992). *Specific speech and language disorders in children.* Whurr, London; Bishop, D., and Mogford, K. (ed.). (1988). *Language development in exceptional circumstances.* Churchill Livingstone, Edinburgh; Wells, G. (1985). *Language development in the pre-school years.* Cambridge University Press.
Law, J. (1992). *The early identification of language development in children.* Chapman & Hall, London.

11. Whitehurst, G.J. and Fischel, J.E. (1994). Practitioner review: early developmental language delay: what, if anything, should the clinician do about it? *Journal of Child Psychology and Psychiatry and Allied Disciplines* 35, 613–48. (A useful overview of intervention for children with language problems, particularly expressive disorders.)

12. Olswang, L.B. and Bain, B.A. (1991). Intervention issues for toddlers with specific language impairments. *Topics in Language Disorders* 11, 69–86.

13. For a comprehensive review of intervention literature, see Enderby, P. and Emerson, J. (1995). *Does speech and language therapy work?* Report to the Department of Health; carried out at Frenchay Hospital, Bristol.

14. The situation is in fact even more complicated, since the SD scores obtained differ according to which test is used.

15. Baron-Cohen, S., Allen, J., and Gillberg, C. (1992). Can autism be detected at 18 months? The needle, the haystack and the CHAT. *British Journal of Psychiatry* 161, 839–43.

16. A group at Strathclyde University have developed a screening test for use in this situation. It has yet to be used extensively under routine working conditions but appears to be based on sound linguistic and psychometric principles: Gillham, B., Boyle, J., Smith, N., and Cheyne, B. (1995). Language screening at 18–36 months: the *First Words* and *First Sentence Tests* and the *First Words Comprehension Cards*. *Child Language Teaching and Therapy* 11, 193–207.

17. Further information on the role of screening for language impairments and the practical problems is being gathered in the Cambridge Language and Speech Project: CLASP.

18. Law, J. (1994). *Before school: a handbook of approaches to intervention with preschool language impaired children.* AFASIC, London (note 8).

19. Ireton, H. (1990). Developmental screening measures. In *Developmental*

assessment in child psychology (ed. J.H. Johnson and J. Goldman), p. 97–8. Pergamon press, New York.

20. Stanovich, K.E. (1994). Does dyslexia exist? *Journal of Child Psychology and Psychiatry* 35, 579–95.

21. For reviews of prevention and intervention, see: Offord, D.R. (1987). Prevention of behavioral and emotional disorders in children. *Journal of Child Psychology and Psychiatry and Allied Disciplines* 28, 9–19.
    Pearce, J. (1993). Child health surveillance for psychiatric disorder: practical guidelines. *Archives of Disease in Childhood* 69, 394–8.
    Stevenson, J. (1990). *Health visitor based services for pre-school children with behavioural problems.* Occasional Paper No. 2, Association for Child Psychology and Psychiatry, London (a collection of papers on health visitor intervention); Nicholl, R. (1993). *Preschool children in troubled families: approaches to intervention and support.* Wiley, Chichester. See also Ireton, note 19.

22. Department of Health (1995). *A handbook on child and adolescent mental health.* Department of Health. Available from HMSO Manchester Print, Logistics Warehouse, Oldham Business Park, Broadgate, Chadderton, Oldham, Lancs OL9 0JA.

23. For recent updates and discussion of the Denver Test see Frankenburg, W.K. (1994). Preventing developmental delays: is developmental screening sufficient? *Pediatrics*, 93, 586–593; Frankenburg, W.K., Dodds, J., Archer, P., Shapiro, H., and Bresnick, B. (1992). The Denver II: a major revision and restandardization of the Denver Developmental Screening Test. *Pediatrics* 89, 91–7.

24. Other tests are discussed by Ireton (note 19) and Meisels, S.J. (1988). Developmental screening in early childhood: the interaction of research and social policy. *Annual Review of Public Health* 9, 527–50.

13

Organization, management, and records

This chapter:

- Emphasizes the need for coordination of child health promotion services
- Proposes how the service might be organized
- Reviews how data should be collected
- Suggests some quality standards
- Notes the increasing problem of litigation
- Summarizes the value and role of personal child health records held by the parent(s)

Introduction

A child health promotion (CHP) programme is a complex undertaking. It involves the primary health care team (as defined on p. 16), a range of specialist services, and other agencies. Ensuring that the service is delivered to every parent is itself a demanding task, but it is even more difficult to monitor quality, measure outcomes, and integrate individual care with public health initiatives.

In the first two editions of *Health for all children* we recommended that one person should be identified in each district to take responsibility for the child health surveillance programme. This suggestion was based on the successful experience with the district immunization coordinator.

A complex task

The need for planning, coordination, and monitoring of all the services involved is as great as ever. However, the task is considerably more complex than we envisaged 5 years ago, for three reasons.

- We have emphasized that the surveillance programme should be seen as just one part of a wider CHP policy.
- The overview of services required in some fields, such as audiology

or ophthalmology, is increasingly sophisticated and calls for a level of expertise likely to be found only in someone with specialist training.

- The emergence of trusts, commissioners, and fund-holders complicates the issue further and makes interagency collaboration more difficult. Some of the tasks outlined below might properly be regarded as provider duties, and others as purchaser responsibilities.

The tasks involved in a successful CHP programme

1. To develop agreed written aims, objectives, referral guidelines, administrative processes, and training standards. This will require coordination of all those involved in CHP, including primary health care staff, paediatricians, public health doctors, nurses, specialists in a variety of fields (audiology, ENT, child development centres, child psychiatry and psychology, etc.), staff of other agencies (education, social services, other local government agencies), and voluntary organizations. All the professionals involved must have the confidence of their colleagues. It is vital that they have a share in 'ownership' of the CHP programme and a mutual interest in its success and effectiveness.

2. To develop and expand targets for coverage and quality standards, and ways of monitoring these.

3. To coordinate training and updating of all staff.

4. To agree criteria and standards required to provide a child health surveillance programme in general practice.

5. To provide advice and information on the CHP programme to purchasing and commissioning authorities, fund-holders, and locality fund-holding groups.

6. To ensure that children who are 'hard to reach' and those 'Looked After' receive the benefits of the CHP programme.

7. To introduce and coordinate new programmes (such as the vitamin K initiative) and to phase out those no longer thought necessary.

8. To establish, develop, and maintain information systems and use these for monitoring, audit, and health services research, and to monitor the issue, maintenance and transfer of child health records (personal child health record).

9. To ensure that the highest standards are maintained in screening programmes, for example for phenylketonuria and hypo-thyroidism, and thereby to protect children from avoidable harm and the health authority and trust from litigation.

10. To prepare both annual and *ad hoc* reports for purchasing and commissioning authorities and to provide information on request for other bodies, such as the Audit Commission, and for voluntary organizations which seek to influence and raise standards in their sphere of interest.

11. To ensure that there is appropriate consultation with parents, children and voluntary groups in the planning and implementation of the programme.

The knowledge and skills required for these tasks are many and varied. They include a knowledge of general and developmental paediatrics, public health, information technology, and community nursing, familiarity with a range of specialized medical fields such as audiology and ophthalmology, experience of general practice, teaching skills, and outstanding organizational and communication ability.

How can this be done? We do not think that it is appropriate for the present Working Party to specify how this should be achieved, but we suggest that the following principles could be agreed:

- There must be close liaison with other groups responsible for child health strategy;
- The range of knowledge and skills listed above is unlikely to be found in one person, and it is more likely that one or more planning or steering groups would be needed;
- Any such group must be multidisciplinary and multi-agency;
- A chairperson should be appointed on a fixed-term basis; this person should be known as the child health promotion coordinator;
- The creation of the planning or steering group(s), the definition of their duties, and the appointment(s) of the individual(s) responsible for these tasks should be a joint undertaking of the commissioning or purchasing authorities (including fund-holding general practitioners) and the provider units;
- The responsibilities of the group(s) and individual(s) should be clearly defined so that questions or concerns about any service or programme can be directed promptly to one person;

- The group(s) should include in its remit an overview of the need for training of all staff. It should also consider the admission of general practitioners to the child health surveillance list and should seek to develop common guidelines with other authorities and with national bodies;
- The group should build on the framework of *Health for all children* in planning its local programme, but the need for flexibility and innovation is stressed.

Data collection

It is neither appropriate nor practical for the Working Party to comment on the type of information system needed in each district or trust,[1] but we propose some guiding principles.

- A database is needed in each district to record details of every live birth. This should form the basis for the monitoring of CHP programmes.
- This common database should be used by all those health care staff with responsibilities for child health.
- It should incorporate a minimum dataset of demographic and birth data, which should be agreed on a national basis.
- It should be able to generate and monitor information, create appointments for immunization and biochemical screening, and measure coverage for specified health reviews (as set out on p. 225).
- The age–sex register maintained by primary health care teams should be used in conjunction with the district database for CHP within individual practices.
- Data should be collected only if they are robust and meaningful. If data are collected on developmental progress or disability, definitions must be unambiguous and interobserver reliability must be high, otherwise the data will be of limited value. (This is difficult to achieve and we question the value of a minimum dataset on these issues until these problems can be resolved.)
- In line with the recommendations of this report, the database should reflect the increased importance of primary prevention and not focus only on the search for defects. For example, data about duration of breast-feeding and administration of vitamin K might be recorded.

- Collection of data on referrals made is of limited value unless the outcome of those referrals can also be ascertained.
- Any CHP information system should be designed to communicate with other databases. For example, linkages with hospital out-patient and admission data, and with accident and emergency attendances, should be possible. The importance of sharing data with social services (e.g. Children Act registers) and with education (e.g. for data on standardized testing) should also be emphasized.
- The system should have the flexibility to permit creation of short-term projects to monitor new interventions or to carry out specific studies. This implies ability either to programme the main data system accordingly or to download from the main dataset to a personal computer.
- The data to be collected should be reflected in medical records and in the personal child health record.
- Parents should be informed about the data system (e.g. through the personal child health record) in line with recent debates about confidentiality and patient data.

Quality checklist

Important adjuncts to successful child health promotion

- Is there a steering group for CHP chaired by a child health promotion coordinator (or some equivalent arrangement)?
- Does this group liaise effectively with a child health strategy group?
- Are there effective referral and follow-up services for 'screen-positive' and 'high-risk' children?
- Are there high-quality services available in response to concerns raised by the primary health care team or parents (general paediatrics, orthopaedics, cardiology, audiology, ophthalmology, nutrition, etc.)?
- Do staff receive training in news-breaking, counselling, and support when serious disorders are suspected?
- Is there an information base about services in the district which is accessible to parents and staff?
- Is home visiting being used sensibly and effectively, for example to

engage families which are hard to reach, support parents with breast-feeding problems, postnatal depression or chronic disability, etc.?

- Is there good liaison and cooperation with other statutory and voluntary agencies? Is there any multi-agency planning forum for children with special needs?

- Is there collaboration between primary health care clinicians, clinical specialists, and public health departments, including an effective information network?

- Is there a multi-agency accident prevention group in the district?

- Has the district appointed an immunization coordinator, a child protection nurse and doctor, and a doctor responsible for liaison with the education authority? Are these individuals allocated sufficient time to carry out their allotted tasks?

- Do contracts specify or recognize time allocated for community development projects?

- Is the personal child health record in use? Is it being used effectively by primary health care team staff and by specialists?

- Is there an information system capable of producing outputs relevant to the needs of professional staff and purchasers? Are any data of doubtful reliability and value being collected?

- Is there an interpreting service for parents whose mother tongue is not English, and a translation facility for written materials?

Specific points to be checked: examples of audit standards

- Immunization and infectious disease prevention (in addition to routine reports on the triple and polio vaccines and *Haemophilus influenza*.
  - Has the 'cold chain' been reviewed?[2]
  - Is there a tuberculosis prevention protocol that defines which babies should receive BCG, aims to ensure that BCG is given to all babies who are eligible before discharge from hospital, describes the arrangements for administering BCG to babies who do not receive it before discharge from hospital, and describes the role of the tuberculosis contact tracer?
  - Do all babies who receive the first dose of hepatitis B vaccine receive the second and third doses as well?
- Is the uptake of phenylketonuria and hypothyroidism testing kept

under review? Are parents told the purpose of the test? Do parents reliably receive results?

- Have services for people with a haemoglobinopathy been reviewed? Has there been any improvement in the service, outcome, and patient satisfaction for people with these conditions?
- Has the maternity unit adopted the Baby Friendly hospital guidelines? Do primary care team staff know about and recommend peer group support for breast-feeding? Do all staff give consistent advice on weaning and dental care?
- Is there an equipment loan store for items needed in injury prevention? Are there arrangements to facilitate safe installation? Do staff know whom to contact when there are obvious hazards needing the attention of housing department officials (e.g. broken balcony railings)?
- Do staff know how to use a depression rating scale? Have they had training in its use and in the management of postnatal depression?
- Does the district use information sheets on reducing the risk of cot death and the hazards of shaking babies?
- Does the district have a choice of options and programmes for supporting parents who need extra help with child rearing?
- Has training been offered for growth monitoring, detection of hearing and vision defects, dislocation of the hip, speech and language disorders, etc.? Do staff have access to a 'Hippy' model for training in hip examinations?
- Does the district meet the audiological service quality standards set out in the document produced by the National Deaf Children's Society?

Litigation

Litigation is an increasing hazard. Missed diagnoses on screening tests are the most obvious example. This would be hard to defend in the case of phenylketonuria or hypothyroidism, but clinical examinations used for screening are well known to be imperfect. It is important that parents are told this. It should not be considered negligent to 'miss' conditions for which no effective screening programme has been identified or recommended in this report. However, it might be negligent not to provide a screening, intervention, or referral service where there is evidence and consensus that this should be done, or to provide a screening service of poor quality which results in diagnoses being missed.

The problems of litigation associated with immunization against pertussis are well known. It should be remembered that an action might also be brought if, for example, a baby contracted tuberculous meningitis because of failure to give BCG or to carry out proper contact tracing, or if an individual developed complications of hepatitis B because of failure to identify or vaccinate a high-risk baby. Examples of other potential causes of legal action include failure to ensure administration of vitamin K, leading to intracranial bleeding, failure to identify hearing loss in the presence of high risk factors, and failure to diagnose reintopathy of prematurity in a high-risk infant.

Personal child health records

This section takes account of the recommendations of the reconvened Working Party on the Personal Child Health Record (Chair, Dr Aidan Macfarlane), set up to revise the record in the light of experience gained over the past three years.[3]

The personal child health record (PCHR) is generally considered to be a successful innovation, and it was in use by more than 75 per cent of districts in England by the end of 1994 and by all four boards in Northern Ireland by early 1995. The procedure for introduction of the PCHR was set out in the first and second editions of *Health for all children*, and is included in this edition as an Appendix.

In addition to improvements in the design and contents (box), a number of issues have been considered by the 1995 Working Party:

When should the record be issued?

There is no universal policy regarding the age at which the record should be issued. The earlier it is given to parents, the more easily it can be used as an adjunct to health information about the child health surveillance programme and as an aid to health promotion. It has been suggested that it should be issued during pregnancy or soon after birth, so that it could be available to record the results of the neonatal examination; however, health visitors do not see every mother during pregnancy (although this is desirable (see page 62), and therefore the task of handing over the record and explaining its use and contents

Use of data for health services monitoring and research It is important to tell parents clearly in the record that the information in the PCHR is computerized and may be used for service and research purposes.

Health promotion data The PCHR should be used to facilitate the health visitor's role in needs assessment and indicate the level of service and degree of priority for CHP agreed with the parents.

Accurate information The information provided in the PCHR should be in line with current recommendations about the content of CHP.

Information about screening The PCHR should emphasize that screening is not 100% perfect and that parents must report any abnormalities—this may give some legal protection in the event of litigation following conditions being 'missed' by screening tests.

PKU and hypothyroidism entries There should be space for positive entry of results rather than the default assumption that no entry means normality.

Injury prevention We propose the use of a developmentally orientated checklist for accident prevention, although the hazards of checklists are well recognized; they are not a substitute for careful counselling and practical advice.

Developmental checklists? We question whether there is a continued need for yes/no checklists for developmental parameters and do not think that there is much value in recording these on a computer database. Developmental information and advice may be given more profitably in other ways.

Charts The PCHR should contain the nine-centile growth charts.
Other information may include:
• benefits information
• the NSPCC 'handle with care' leaflet which can be used as a non-threatening way of discussing child abuse with any parent
• the FSID leaflet *Reducing the risk,* which simplifies discussion of cot death and preventive measures
• Information about services for special needs children
• Lists of risk factors for hearing loss and vision defects.

would largely be the responsibility of midwives. Concern has been expressed about distress to the parents in the event of intrapartum death or stillbirth, but we suggest that in these circumstances the parents would value the record as part of their memory of the baby they lost.

Health Education Authority publications

The Health Education Authority publication *From birth to five* should be given to every first-time mother and used in conjunction with the PCHR.

Language and ethnic issues

Translations of the PCHR or at least of the key pages would be valued by members of ethnic minorities, but the need should be assessed in each district and for each ethnic group. A library of translations should be maintained to reduce duplication of labour.[4]

Handing the record to the child

The PCHR should be passed on to the child when leaving school and should accompany them if they are 'Looked After' or adopted.

Should the record be used in school?

There are a number of practical problems to be solved in using the PCHR in school and these have yet to be resolved.

Ownership

The information in the record belongs to the parent, although technically the record itself, the physical object, belongs to the Secretary of State.

Duplicate records

Most primary health care staff find that it is necessary to keep some duplicate records. In most cases, these should be kept to a minimum and need record only the timing of visits, contacts, and reviews, together with essential data such as measurements and immunizations. More detailed records may be needed about complex problems or child protection concerns. It is generally agreed that openness with parents is essential. Staff keeping their own notes should remember that all professional records may be seen by parents if they so request. The PCHR can only play a role in developing true partnership between parents and professionals if information and opinions are shared.

Notes and references

A more extensive bibliography is available on personal child health records; see p. xi for details.

1. For a review of the technical aspects of information needs: Blair, M. (1995). NHS information strategy and its impact on child health. *Archives of Disease in Childhood* 72, 355–7.
2. See Thakker, Y. and Woods, S. (1992). Storage of vaccines in the community: weak link in the cold chain? *British Medical Journal* 304, 756–8.
3. The most recent overview of the use of Personal Child Health Records will be found in Saffin, K. (1994) (ed.). *Where now? What next? Personal Child Health Records. Proceedings of the national meeting held in Oxford on September 14th 1994.* Available from Mrs Sheila Halliday, Oxfordshire Community NHS Trust, Bourton House, 18 Thorney Leys Park, Witney, Oxon OX8 7GE (Price £12.75 incl. p. & p.)
4. A library of pages created for the Personal Child Health Record is maintained; before developing new pages, it is worth checking to see if it has already been done: contact the PCHR library, British Paediatric Association, 5 St Andrews Place, Regents Park, London NW1 4LB.

14

Summary of 1995 child health promotion programme

Introduction

At first sight, the programme outlined here has not changed very much, except in points of detail, from that set out in the first two editions of *Health for all children*. However, we wish to emphasize a number of points which, if accepted, imply substantial changes in the approach to preventive child health services.

Terminology We have suggested that child health promotion (CHP) is a more suitable title for the programme as a whole. Child health surveillance (CHS) is part of the programme and refers specifically to secondary prevention by early detection. Currently, general practitioners are contracted to provide a CHS service, rather than health promotion. Nevertheless, it is vital that both health promotion and CHS are regarded as the tasks of the whole primary health care team. Some aspects of CHS may best be carried out by health visitors, whereas health education given by doctors at appropriate times may be very effective. In due course, it will be important to consider whether contracts should be broader based, encompassing child health promotion rather than CHS in isolation.

More emphasis on primary prevention In focusing on aspects of health promotion, we have stressed that more resources could be devoted to primary prevention. This should begin in pregnancy or, better still, before conception, for example by personal, social, and health education in schools. It is important that midwives and other members of the primary health care team collaborate closely.

A more coordinated and determined effort should be made to address topics such as accident prevention, good nutrition, dental care, and postnatal depression. The advice given by health professionals to individual parents should be in line with the overall policy for the whole community. Accident prevention, nutrition, and dental prophylaxis are examples of topics on which a detailed local policy should be developed. Unless there are good reasons to the contrary, these should conform closely to national guidelines.

Better referral arrangements We have emphasized, more strongly than before, the vital importance of planning CHS in conjunction with the colleagues who will receive referrals when abnormalities are suspected. Primary health care teams responsible for providing CHS services should insist on clear guidelines for referral and should monitor the quality of service and the waiting time experienced by their patients.

More emphasis on collaboration between health services and other agencies Arrangements must be negotiated with education and social services for the provision of developmental guidance and support to families with special needs or problems, and to ensure that the prevention and follow-up of child abuse is maintained at a satisfactory standard. The value of the services provided by voluntary agencies and the role of lay workers, although needing further research, are emphasized.

The need to 'target' services The evidence reviewed in Chapter 2 suggests that the aims of health promotion are broadly similar for most families, but the need for professional input to help parents achieve them varies widely. Positive discrimination in favour of families with complex needs is necessary. This implies that, unless resources are increased, many families will receive a reduced level of service. Flexibility, greater trust in the judgement of front-line clinical staff, and a less prescriptive approach on the part of service planners and managers are essential if these aims are to be fulfilled.

Fewer screening procedures The number of procedures which in our view fulfil the criteria for screening tests is even smaller than recommended previously.

More flexibility There is correspondingly more scope for flexibility in deciding how best to ensure that the aims of the health promotion programme can be accomplished. The aim of the programme should be equity of outcome, but this does not imply or need equity of input.

More confident recommendations In several instances, accumulating evidence has encouraged the Working Party to make recommendations with greater confidence than was justified in the first and second editions of *Health for all Children.*

The importance of the personal child health record (PCHR) and the Health Education Authority book *Birth to five* as health education tools is stressed.

The core surveillance programme for individual children

The following summary of the recommended programme incorporates details of the specified health checks, gives examples of topics for health education at different ages, and stresses the importance of record systems that facilitate communication, clinical audit, and epidemiological monitoring. Some health promotion topics are relevant to all families and should be regarded as part of the core programme. Examples include immunization and advice about reducing the risk of cot death.

Care in the first few weeks of life is particularly important. No one pattern of working can be described as the ideal, but it is essential that midwives, health visitors, and general practitioners agree on the arrangements within each practice so that families are neither overvisited nor neglected.

Records and information transfer After each review, information should be passed to the appropriate authority or agency (FHSA/DHA, district or community offices, etc.) to facilitate monitoring for the individual child and for the district as a whole.

Education Act and the 1994 Code of Practice The responsibilities of NHS staff set out by this legislation (see p. 79 for details) should be remembered at each of the regular reviews described below. The fact that this is normal procedure should be made clear to parents; preferably it should also be stated in the PCHR.

Neonatal examination

This is usually the responsibility of hospital staff, but may be performed by the general practitioner in the case of home deliveries, babies born in general practitioner obstetric units, and very early (less than 6 hours) discharges. With the increasing role of midwives as independent practitioners, it may well be the midwife who has the initial responsibility for assessing the newborn infant and identifying any congenital abnormalities.

The advice given below reflects the trend to earlier discharge of infants after birth. This means that it will be increasingly common for serious congenital abnormalities to present after the infant has gone home. The training of primary health care staff must be updated accordingly.

The neonatal examination consists of:

Review of family history, pregnancy and birth, and of any concerns expressed by parents. Physical examination including weight and head circumference. Note and discuss any birthmarks. Check for cyanosis and tachypnoea. Note that absence of a murmur does not exclude heart defects and that serious congenital heart disease may present at any time in the early weeks of life. Check for congenital dislocation of hips (CDH) and testicular descent. Inspect eyes. View red reflux of fundus with ophthalmoscope (for cataract) but do not attempt fundoscopy. If high-risk category for hearing defect, consider EOAE or BSER* test of hearing (and if personal child health record has been issued, show parents check list of advice for detection of hearing loss). PKU and thyroid tests to be done at usual time. Haemoglobinopathy screen if specified in local policy.

Topics for Health Education

Explain to the parents that a normal neonatal examination is not a guarantee that the infant will have no problems and ensure that they feel free to obtain advice at once if concerned. Emphasize advice about reducing the risk of cot death. Discuss the following as appropriate: feeding and nutrition, vitamin K, baby care, sibling management, crying and sleep problems, and transport in cars.

First two weeks

The health visitor carries out a first visit to all families, usually when the baby is around 10–14 days old. This is used to establish contact (if this had not been done during pregnancy) and to start assessing the probable health care needs of that family.

* OAE (otoacoustic emissions) and BSER (brainstem-evoked response) are the two methods of testing the hearing which are most likely to be used for screening neonates.

Many general practitioners consider it good practice to see all new babies soon after delivery, whether or not they are carrying out the formal neonatal examination. This provides an opportunity to evaluate any concerns raised by the parents, and to cement the relationship with the family. In addition to the immediate benefits, this contact can be the prelude to an effective programme of surveillance and helps the members of the primary health care team to estimate the level of support and assistance that each new parent is likely to require.

Further physical examination should be undertaken if appropriate. If available, details of the neonatal examination help in deciding what is needed; items omitted at the neonatal examination, for whatever reason, should be carried out. Signs that might indicate heart disease (p. 96) should be sought and taken seriously. Provided that the hips were checked during the neonatal examination, and the result has been recorded, it is not essential to repeat this (p. 94).

Topics for health education

(NB Some of these topics may be deferred until the 6–8-week examination and review). Nutrition and breast-feeding (including peer support); check need for further dose of vitamin K and whether it has been supplied and/or given; parental smoking; accident prevention—bathing, scalding by feeds, fires. Immunization—this should include determining if the baby is eligible for BCG and if so whether it has been given, and also whether the baby will need follow-up doses of hepatitis B vaccine. Reason for and results of PKU and thyroid tests (and discuss haemoglobinopathy if indicated)—remind parents to request results of these tests and ensure that they are noted in the record. Significance of prolonged jaundice. Depression is common—how to cope and obtain help. Offer help with benefits review if relevant.

Six to eight weeks

This examination should be undertaken by a member of the primary health care team responsible for the child's surveillance. It is usually done by a doctor; the presence of the health visitor facilitates the sharing and follow-up of any anxieties, particularly with regard to feeding problems, depression, etc. A health visitor could learn to undertake this examination and carry out the specified checks, but we are not aware of any detailed reports on the benefits and disadvantages of this arrangement.

The examination may be undertaken at the same visit as the first immunization and/or the postnatal check for the mother; this is a matter for individual teams to decide. It consists of:

*Check history and ask about parental concerns. Physical examination, weight, and head circumference. Measure length if indicated. Check for CDH and, if in doubt, refer **urgently**. If testes not descended, arrange referral (p. 106). Prolonged jaundice should have been identified earlier—if found at this review, refer immediately. Enquire particularly about concerns regarding vision and hearing. Inspect eyes. Do not attempt hearing test. If a high-risk hearing screening service is provided, check again whether baby in high-risk category for hearing loss and refer if necessary. Discuss immunization; record whether or not there is any contraindication; signed consent is **not** essential, but should be obtained at this visit if thought desirable by individual practitioners or required by locally agreed protocols. Address any outstanding topics not covered from the list suggested for health education for the first 2 weeks.*

Topics for health education
Immunization; feeding, nutrition; weaning (explain about doorstep milk and iron deficiency); reinforce sudden infant death syndrome advice; smoking, postnatal depression; dangers of fires, falls, overheating, and scalds; recognition of illness in babies and what to do; how to use NHS facilities effectively.

Two, three, and four months

The baby should receive the primary course of immunizations at these ages. No specific checks are required, but the parent should have the opportunity to discuss any concerns with the appropriate member of the primary health care team. Some districts may opt to recheck the hips at the same time as the third immunization.

Weighing in the first six months
Regular weighing of normal healthy babies is of uncertain value (p. 112). There is no doubt that parents value this procedure because of the reassurance it gives them that all is well, but health professionals should be aware of both the unnecessary anxiety and the false sense of security it can provide.

Facilities for weighing should be available as part of a CHS service. There is no reason why the parents should not weigh the baby themselves if they so wish.

Six to nine months

This examination can be undertaken by the doctor and health visitor together, or it can be regarded as primarily the health visitor's responsibility. There is no reason why the health visitor should not learn to check the hips.

The age of 6–9 months was selected because this is the ideal time for the distraction test of hearing. However, this should be done in protected time and there is no specific reason why the other aspects of this review should be done within this age band. For example, it could be carried out at the same time as the MMR vaccine (13 months). However, we stress that, as far as we are aware, this possibility has not been investigated in practice.

Enquire about parental concerns regarding health and development. Ask specifically about vision and hearing. Check weight if parents request or if indicated. Measure length if indicated. Look for evidence of CDH (but see above). Observe visual behaviour and look for squint. Carry out distraction test of hearing or other procedures as agreed with FHSA. NB **Two** *adequately trained staff are required for this test.*

Topics for health education
Accident prevention: choking; scalds and burns; falls; drowning risk in bath; anticipate increasing mobility, i.e. safety gates, guards, etc. Nutrition: emphasize problem of iron deficiency and how to prevent it. Smoking. Review of transport in cars. Dental prophylaxis. Developmental needs. Sunburn.

Thirteen months

MMR vaccine.

Eighteen to twenty-four months

This review is probably more usefully carried out as close to 24 months as possible, since some aspects, notably height and language acquisition, are more readily assessed in the slightly older child. It does not involve any specific medical or screening procedures, and is concerned primarily with parent guidance and education. It is often carried out at the family home and it is suggested that the health visitor is the most appropriate person to take responsibility for this examination. The place where this is done, and the amount of time devoted to this review in each case, should be decided on the basis of the primary health care team's overall knowledge of the child and family. The content of the review is as follows.

Enquire about parental concerns, particularly regarding behaviour, vision, and hearing. Confirm that child is walking with normal gait. Explain why comprehension (understanding when spoken to) and interest in social communication are more important at this age than speech production. Absence or small number of words at this age is not cause for serious concern. Formal tests of language are not recommended as a routine but may be used by appropriately trained individuals if in doubt or to demonstrate points to a parent. Parents should be counselled and follow-up arranged if there is any reason for concern or if the parent wishes. Do not attempt formal screening tests of vision or hearing. Arrange detailed assessment if in doubt. Remember high prevalence of iron deficiency anaemia at this age. Carry out haemoglobin estimation if local policy. Measure height (NB If this review is carried out by telephone or post, as suggested by some health visitors when the parent is experienced and has no worries, it is important to ensure that height and gait are checked on an opportunistic basis. It is in any case good practice to measure height whenever a child visits the surgery or clinic (see p. 119 for explanation).

Topics for health education
Accident prevention: falls from heights including windows; drowning; poisoning; road safety. Smoking. Developmental needs; language and play. Benefits of mixing with other children—playgroup etc. Avoidance and management of behaviour problems.

Review at 3¼–3½ years

The aims are to ensure that the child is physically fit and that there are no medical disorders or defects which may interfere with education, to ensure that the immunizations are up to date, and to determine whether there are problems with development, language, or behaviour which may have educational implications.

For many families, this review will be very brief. The majority of children with significant developmental problems have already been identified by this age and the proportion will increase if nursery education becomes the norm. A particular effort may be needed to review children who are not in any nursery facility, attend a child-minder, and are persistent non-attenders for immunizations etc. It is among this group that one is most likely to find children with potentially serious developmental problems which might otherwise be overlooked.

We recommend that (a) each primary care team should decide whether this review should be performed by a doctor or a health visitor, since it no longer contains any screening procedure which calls for physical examination skills, and (b) flexibility and judgement should be exercised in deciding how much time to devote to this review for each family, depending on the team's knowledge of the child, frequency of other contacts, etc.

Part or all of the review can be done in combination with the preschool booster. (The latter can be given at any time once 3 years have elapsed from the last of the three primary immunizations.)*

The review consists of:

*Enquiry and discussion about vision, squint, hearing, behaviour, language acquisition, and development. Be aware of the agreed indications for referral, particularly with respect to speech and language problems. If there are any concerns, discuss with the parent whether the child is likely to have any special educational problems or needs and arrange further action as appropriate. Ensure that the specialist paediatric services are informed if there is **any** anxiety about a child's education potential (see p. 79). Measure height and plot on chart. Weigh if indicated. Check for testicular descent only if there is no previous note in the personal child health record. Carry out physical examination if indicated, for example because of any physical complaint or if child appears not to have had any recent medical assessment for some other reason (e.g. newly arrived in the UK). If concerned about possible hearing impairment, perform hearing test **if** adequately trained and equipped; otherwise refer. Vision screening is of doubtful value unless performed by a trained person, usually an*

---

* This is the usual recommendation, but we know of no scientific reason why it need be observed rigidly.

*orthoptist. It is **not** recommended that doctors or health visitors should do this.*

Topics for Health Education

Accidents: fires, roads, drowning. Begin to teach road safety. Preparation for school. Nutrition and dental care.

Five years (school entry—range approximately 54–66 months)

The school entrant medical examination is usually undertaken by the staff of the school health service rather than by primary health care teams (see the Polnay Report (note 3, p. 107)).

Some authorities believe that *all* school entrants should be offered not only a physical examination but also a full developmental evaluation. However, in many districts and boards, the universal 'cohort' examination of all school entrants has been discontinued because the yield of new abnormalities is small. Only selected children are examined, on the basis of previously inadequate or poorly documented preschool surveillance, or concerns raised by parents or teachers.

Whichever policy is adopted, it seems likely that a well-conducted preschool surveillance programme, as outlined above, will progressively reduce the need for, and the yield of, detailed school entrant examinations.

Nevertheless, the following are recommended for *all* children as a minimum at school entry:

Enquire about parental and teacher concerns. Review preschool records. Measure height and plot on chart. Check vision using Snellen chart. Check hearing by 'sweep' test.

In many schools these checks are combined in a health interview in which the opportunity is taken to provide health education relevant to school health. The school nurse may be solely responsible for this task or may share it with the school doctor.

Appendix 1

Third Joint Working Party on Child Health Surveillance Membership, Observers, Contributors and Critical Friends

Professor D. M. B. Hall (*Chairman*)   British Paediatric Association
Dr A. MacFarlane   British Paediatric Association
Dr M. Miles   British Paediatric Association
Dr. D. Sowden   Royal College of General Practitioners
Ms K. Billingham   Royal College of Nursing
Ms J. Naish   Royal College of Nursing
Dr G. Emrys Jones   General Medical Services Committee of the British Medical Association
Ms S. Botes   Health Visitors' Association
Dr A. Waterston   British Association for Community Child Health
Dr S. Stewart-Brown   Faculty of Public Health Medicine
Ms K. Ford   Health Education Authority
Dr D. Ernaelsteen, Dr H. Williams   Observers, Department of Health
Dr A. Findlay   Observer, Scottish Home & Health Department
Dr J. Richards   Observer, NHS Executive
Dr Heideh Shahsavan   Observer, World Health Organization
Professor J. Butler   Critical Friend, Health Services Research Unit, University of Kent
Dr B. Mayall   Critical Friend, The Social Science Research Unit, Institute of Education
Professor G. Lindsay   Critical Friend, Dept. of Educational Psychology, University of Sheffield
Dr J. Andrews   Observer, Welsh Office
Dr P. Woods   Observer, Department of Health & Social Services, Northern Ireland
Ms M. Blackburn   Co-opted Member
Ms Buxton   Co-opted Member
Ms J. Waterfield   Co-opted Member
Ms. C. Brummel   Co-opted Member
Ms J. Morgan   Co-opted Member
Dr S. Kendall   Co-opted Member

Appendix 2

Parent-held records

There is an increasing weight of opinion that parents should hold the child's main record. Recent legislation implies that parents will have an increasing right to examine their child's medical records, and parents are no more likely to lose the record than are professionals.

If held by parents, the record is available for consultation to any professional involved with the child. Further, parent-held records are in keeping with the philosophy that parents should be treated as equal partners in child health care.

We conclude that the parent-held record is a desirable development and one that should be supported. Nevertheless, we recognize the need for some information to be held by health professionals. This must include personal information, a note as to whether the agreed health surveillance checks and immunizations have been carried out, and if so the dates and the outcome. These details should be in a form in which they can readily be entered into a computer record system. There must also be space for clinical notes, the names of people to whom referrals have been made and the outcome, and the information required for overall monitoring.

We are not enthusiastic about the idea of a detailed developmental record chart for each child. We would see this as a continuation of the 'box ticking' approach to developmental screening, which we believe to be outdated. In cases where a child's development gives cause for concern a developmental record may be very useful, but is likely to be more profitable when it forms part of an intervention programme.

Editorial comment

The working party on parent-held records has now published its recommendations and the Personal Child Health Record (PCHR) is available for purchase. The concept has been widely supported by all the professional bodies concerned and is welcomed by consumer representatives. Preliminary reports are favourable. Several individuals are now considering the issue of translating the PCHR into other languages, but this will need to be addressed at national level for reasons of economy.

A number of points need further consideration by districts or boards planning to introduce the PCHR, and it may be useful to reproduce here the advice offered in some districts and boards regarding the introduction of the PCHR.

1. *One person should take responsibility* for the introduction of the PCHR. This person will usually be the doctor or nurse with overall responsibility for the Community Child Health service, or someone delegated by him/her.

2. The concept and advantages of the PCHR should be *discussed with community doctors and nurses*, and with paediatric staff in the hospital department of paediatrics/child health. It may be appropriate to raise the matter at relevant meetings; for example, the Divisions of Child Health and of Obstetrics and Gynaecology. A commitment to the introduction of the PCHR should be established. *A small working group* should be set up to implement the introduction of the new record.

3. The support of the *local FHSA* should be obtained, followed by an approach to all *local GPs*, using whatever channels are recommended by the FHSA managers.

4. A source of *funding* for the PCHR should be identified. *Stocks of existing records should be run down* and instructions given to the Supplies department about re-ordering of existing records and the proposed date of introduction of the PCHR. The *savings made* from the phasing out of existing records should be calculated.

5. The working group should consider whether any *local information* is to be included in the Record, and whether any *modification* to the National format are required in the light of local conditions. For example, a page may be needed to explain the details of a neonatal hearing screening programme. Some GPs have prepared an information page about their practice, to be inserted in the PCHR.

6. The group will need to consider how *surveillance information is to be transferred* from GPs to the Health Authority (as required by the New Contract). One option offered in the PCHR is the use of non-carbon copies of routine surveillance reports which can be sent direct to the Community or FHSA offices for computer data entry. These record forms may need modification to make them compatible with local computer requirements. Clerical staff in clinics and GP premises will need to know the arrangements for transferring information to the central monitoring office.

There is a growing body of opinion that parents should know about the maintenance of a community record system required for monitoring and also about any special registers such as those kept about childen with Special Educational Needs. A page containing information of local relevance about such matters can be inserted into the PCHR; this would meet the concerns expressed by many health professionals regarding the transfer of information and the perceived threat to confidentiality posed by information technology.

7. *Orders should be placed* for the number of records required and for any additional printing needed for local additions. The order should specify whether or not non-carbon copies are to be included on the surveillance report forms.

8. A decision must be made about the best way of *handing the PCHR to the parent*. Most districts will probably decide that the health visitor's first home visit after the baby's birth is the optimum time for this. Other options are to issue it in the postnatal ward, or even to present it to mothers attending antenatal classes. In Districts where there is substantial cross-boundary flow, it may be necessary to make arrangements with neighbouring health authorities regarding the issue of, and payment for, the PCHR.

9. Some Health Authorities may wish to provide each parent with a copy of the *neonatal discharge summary*, to be filed in the PCHR; and some Neonatal Intensive Care Units may also follow this practice. Discussion with the Department of Obstetrics may be required.

10. Although it is essential that all staff should regard the PCHR as the child's main surveillance record, a *professional record* will still be needed. Health visitors and clinic doctors will need to record that routine contacts have taken place; major problems and concerns must be summarized; health visitors will wish to continue their practice of keeping family records together. It is not desirable to perpetuate the practice of having separate records for doctors and health visitors, or for pre-school and school-age children.

Accordingly, the working group will need to decide on the format of a *Common Professional Record*, which can be used by *all* community health care staff. The storage of and access to these professional records will also have to be decided, both for children whose surveillance is offered by their GP and for those who remain the responsibility of the Community Child Health Service.

11. The working group may wish to consider whether the PCHR is to be used for the *maintenance of a record of therapy* in the case of children with chronic diseases; for example, asthma, diabetes, severe handicapping conditions, or epilepsy. They may also wish to ensure that for children with disorders that affect growth, such as Turner's and Down's syndromes, *special growth charts* are supplied.

12. Since the PCHR contains some pages devoted to *Health Education*, a policy for the use of this and other Health Education publications and materials should be developed.

13. *Training sessions* will be required to introduce the concept of the PCHR to medical and nursing staff. While some doctors now give copies of summaries, reports, and letters to parents, this is still the exception rather than the rule. Staff will need to consider issues of openness and honesty, sharing information, parent involvement in decision-making, and confidentiality. In particular, the use of the PCHR in cases of concern about *child abuse or neglect* will need to be addressed, preferably in a joint training session with social services.

The issues involved with the PCHR in this situation are related to those raised by the attendance of parents at case conferences; this is similarly an important topic for continuing education. Managers must allocate sufficient time for continuing education.

Index

Note: page numbers in *italics* refer to figures and tables

abduction 70
accidents, *see* injury, unintentional
achondroplasia 123
adrenal hyperplasia, congenital
    115
advice, quality 19–20
advocacy 12
air pollution 102
amblyopia 165, 167–8, 176
    detection 168
anaemia
    thalassaemia 134
    see also iron deficiency anaemia
aphasia 180
    acquired receptive 186
Asperger's syndrome 190–1
assessment 202
asthma 101–2
    physical examination 106
    primary prevention 101–2
    smoking 106
atlanto–axial subluxation in Down's
    syndrome 136, 138
atrial septal defects 98–9
attachment behaviour 67
attentional deficit 206
audiological programmes 162
audiology service 5, 158, 218
    coordinator 159–60
audiometry, pure tone 156
audit 2, 18
    audiological programmes 162
    growth monitoring 124
auditory agnosia 186
auditory response cradle 153
autism *181*, 190–1
autistic spectrum disorder 190–1,
    206

baby blues 63
Baby Friendly Initiative 52
balance in otitis media with effusion
    148
BCG vaccination 42, 217
    litigation 219
behaviour
    attachment 67
    difficulties 7
    disorders 179–208
    examination at 3¼–3½ years 231
    health-related 29
    home environment assessment 203
    iron deficiency anaemia 140–1
    otitis media with effusion 148
    parental concerns 33, 230
    parental support/advice 3
    screening concept 199–203
behavioural problems 67–8
    education professionals liaison 68
    identification 198
    mild 196–9
    with vision impairment 165
biliary atresia, extrahepatic 135
biotinidase deficiency 132
blood pressure screening 100–1, 105–6
body mass index charts 121, 125
bone dysplasia 111
brain-stem evoked response audiometry
    153
    neonatal tests 226
breastfeeding 51
    intention 51
    lactation establishment 51–2
    maintenance 52
    otitis media with effusion protection
        147
brain injury, acquired 181

Cambridge crowding cards 169
cardiovascular system examination 98
care of next infant 57
cataract 164
cerebral palsy
    acquired hip disorders 96
    disability 180, *181*
    early detection 78
    neonatal encephalopathy 182
child abuse 33
    language development 186
    mental health of mother 63
    parental awareness 6
    prevention 68–70
    risk 22
        factors 68, 69
    secondary prevention 70
    weight gain 113
Child Health Promotion 1
    community-based projects 13
    goals 2
    health care needs identification 3
    partnerships 3
    Programme 17
        coordinator 7, 214
        policy statement 7
    services 2
    surveillance 9
    tasks 2
    see also health promotion
child health service, evidence-based
        16–17
child protection 68–70
Children Act (1989) 79, 206
    children in need 22
circumcision 102
cleft palate
    otitis media with effusion 147
    speech impairment 194
clinical interventions 13
clinics, access 37
clumsiness 180, 184, 195
coarctation 99
cochlear implantation 150
Code of Practice (1994) 225
coeliac disease 136, 138
cognitive deficit 186

environmental deprivation 206
cold chain 217
colour vision defects 173, 175–6, 177
commissioning authorities 213
communication
    deaf children 150
    disorders 206
    examination at eighteen to
        twenty-four months 230
    impairment 6, 190–1
    interprofessional 183, 184
    professional-parent 207
    structured groups 65
community
    development 12
    paediatric nursing services 20
    profiling 34
community-based projects 13
comprehension
    deficit 190, 191
    examination at eighteen to
        twenty-four months 230
conditional reference 127
    charts 114
confidentiality 216
constitutional delay in growth and
        puberty 115
consumer information 13
consumerism pressures 32
core programme
    immunizations 18
    reviews/checks 27
    routine reviews 18
cot death, *see* sudden infant death
        syndrome
counselling 23–5
    child abuse 70
    early diagnosis 78
    genetic 78
    sickle cell disease 134
    see also genetic counselling
cow's milk, unmodified 140, 143, 144
cranial irradiation 111
craniostenosis 125
crowding phenomenon 169
cystic fibrosis 132
    diagnostic tests/screening 137

cytomegalovirus *147*
    sensorineural hearing loss 151

database 215–16
deaf community 150
defect detection 1
dental caries 54
    fluoride 55
dental disease 54–7
    nutritional advice 55
    primary prevention 56–7
    prophylaxis 58
dental erosion 54, 56
Denver Developmental Screening test
        201
depression 36
    intervention 64
    loneliness 64–5
    mothers 63
    postnatal 63, 227
    prevention 63–4
    rating scale 218
    reactive 63
deprivation 31
    environmental 195, 206
    language development 186
    learning disabilities 195
    middle-class parents 33
    social 198–9
detection, early 77–8, 77–9
    6–8 week examinations 79
    congenital heart disease 96–7
    congenital hip dislocation 93
    hearing defects 149–58
    neonatal 79
    neurological illness 79–80
    opportunist 81
    outcome 78
    quality of life 78
    vision impairment 164–5
    see also diagnosis
development
    assessment
        effectiveness 204
        home environment 203
        for school entrants 203–4

checklists 220
delay 206
disorders 179–208
examination 202, 231
impairment
    adverse prognostic significance
        206–7
    educational support 207
    unpredictability 200
intervention programmes 70–3
iron deficiency anaemia 140–1
mental health of mother 63–5
parental support/advice 3
promoting 61–74
testing 6
visual 174
developmental screening 202
    concept 199–203
    effectiveness 204
    programmes 205
    questionnaires 201
    tests 201
diagnosis
    missed 131, 218–19
    see also detection, early
diet
    cultural resistance 110
    unusual 58
dieticians 25
disability 36, 179–80
    assessment services 207
    causes *181*
    conditions 180
    helping children 206
    high-prevalence low-severity 180,
        184, *185*, 186–9, 186–99
        language acquisition 184, *185*,
            186–94
        speech 184, *185*, 186–94
    identifying children 206
    low-prevalence high-severity
        conditions 180, 180–4
        communication with parents
            183
        detection 182
        evolutionary diagnoses 183
        high-risk follow-up 182–3

disability (*cont.*)
  low-prevalence high-severity
    conditions (*cont.*)
    management 183–4
      parental input 183
    management services 207
    referral 207
    terminology 15
disease prevention 13–14, 217
  see also infectious disease
distraction screening test 5, 154–5,
    160–1
  economics 155–6
  examination at six to nine months
    229
Down's syndrome
  atlanto–axial subluxation 136, 138
  congenital heart disease 97, 105
  growth charts 123
  hypothyroidism 131
    screening 6
  otitis media with effusion 147
  thyroid disorders 137
Duchenne muscular dystrophy 78, 133,
    181
  disability *181*
  walking age 195
dyslexia 175, 184, 195
dysmorphic syndromes 174
dysphasia 181

eating problems 58
Edinburgh Postnatal Depression Scale
    64
education
  early intervention 71
  investment 11
  materials 37
  special needs 78–9, 231
Education Act (1993) 79, 206, 225
emotional difficulties 67–8, 179
  environmental deprivation 206
encephalopathy, neonatal 182
endocarditis predisposition 97
endocrine deficiency disorders 115
environmental deprivation

  adverse effects 206
  language impairment 195
  learning disabilities 195
ethnic groups
  family's mother tongue 191
  interpreting service 217
  needs 25
  personal child health record
    translations 221
evaluation 2
evoked otoacoustic emissions 151,
    153–4
  neonatal tests 226
eyes, neonatal examination 174

facial malformation syndromes 147
failure to thrive 112, 113
  congenital heart disease 98
  growth monitoring 124
  non-organic 5, 113
  thalassaemia 134
familial large head 125
families
  at risk 32–3
  high risk 22
  individual health promotion needs
    34–6
  needs 31
    assessment 34–5, 37
    determination 3, 36
  poverty 31–2
  relationships 198
  spacing 181
  support 3, 20
  vulnerable 22
fathers 30
  involvement 37
feeding difficulties 113
financial benefits 11
fluoride 55
folic acid supplementation 181
fund-holders 213

gait 95, 104, 230
galactosaemia 132

general practitioner 225, 227
genetic counselling 78, 181
  heart disease 98
genitalia
  abnormalities 102
  ambiguous 102
genital mutilation, female 70
Glasgow acuity cards 169
glaucoma 164
grommets 149
growth
  constitutional delay 115
  disorder identification 121
  impairment 111
  iron supplementation effects
    143
  slow *124*
growth charts 116, *120*
  children with disabilities 123
  interpretation 122
  nine-centile 116, *120*
growth hormone insufficiency
    115
  growth monitoring 111
  late-onset 121
  weight gain 112
growth monitoring 5, 109–28
  accuracy 118
  audit 124
  benefits 110–12
  disorder detection 110
  effective 116–19, *120*, 121
  growth impairment 111
  head circumference 125–7
  health promotion 110
  length measurement 114
  measurement techniques 116, 117,
    119
  public health 110
  regression to the mean 127–8
  reproducibility 118
  research 124–5
  in schools 125
  screening 109
  short-term variability 118
  value 109–10
  weight 112–14

haematoma 125
haemoglobin levels 140, 142, 144
haemoglobinometer 142
haemoglobinopathies 6, 134–5, 226
  screening 137–8
handicap terminology *15*
hardship, personal 32
head circumference 125–7
  measurement 126–7
head injury prevention 181
Health Alliances 11, 37
health care needs
  assessment 3, 22–3
    barriers 23
  child perceptions 23
  determination 21–2
  individual 22–3
  unmet 23
health education 12–13
  topics 226, 227, 228, 229, 230, 232
Health Education Authority
    publications 220
Health of the Nation smoking target 44
health professionals
  advice to parents 81–2
  health promotion skills 29
  intuition 22
  multi-agency planning 214, 217
  needs assessment 23
  sensitivity requirements 82
  see also paraprofessionals
health promotion 9–10, 19–37
  adverse outcomes 29
  aims 20
  benefits 30
  checklists 22
  community level 34
  counselling 23–5
  data 220
  defined 10
  disciplines involved 28
  effectiveness 30–3
  ethical considerations 27–8
  ethnic groups needs 25
  evaluation 28–30
  father influence 30
  flexibility of delivery 36

health promotion (*cont.*)
  geographic areas 34
  growth monitoring 110
  hazards 35–6
  individual families 34–6
  input levels 29
  interventions 10
  leaflets 25
  literacy 25
  management systems 37
  monitoring 29, 37
  needs assessment 21
  non-qualified staff 26
  outcome measures 28
  parental responsibility 19
  preventive model 10–11
  public policy 11
  research 37
  resource allocation 37
  responsibility 20–1
  self-empowerment model 11
  service profile 28–9
  skills of professionals 29
  society's interest 19
  socio-economic factors 10–11
  support 23–5
  surveillance 27
  targeting 33–6
  tasks 21–7
  written information 25
  see also Child Health Promotion
health promotion programme 222–32
  audit standards 217–18
  consultation 214
  coordination 212–13
  core surveillance programme 225–32
  data collection 215–16
  domestic safety 218
  information base 216, 217
  information system 217
  inter-agency collaboration 224
  interpreting service 217
  monitoring 212–13
  personal child health records 225
  planning 212–13
    groups 214–15
  primary prevention 222–3

quality checklist 216–18
  referral 223
  reports 214
  screening procedures 224
  service targeting 224
  staff training 216, 218
  steering groups 214–15, 216
  successful 30, *31*
  tasks 213–15
  terminology 223
health protection 11
health records 213
health surveillance, *see* surveillance
health visitors 20–1
  examination at six to eight weeks
    227
  examination at six to nine months
    229
  health care need determination 21–1
  identification of psychological
    problems 199
  intensive programmes 71
hearing
  aid *147*, 149
  behaviour 191
  examination at 3¼–3½ years 231
  examination at five years 232
  parental concerns 230
  screening 5
  test at six to nine months 229
hearing defects/loss 146–9
  acquired 159
  behavioural testing 154
  causes *147*
  conductive 146–9
  congenital 85
    sensorineural 78, 149
  distraction screening test 5, 154–6,
    160–1, 229
  dual pathology 155
  early diagnosis 149–58
  early intervention 161
  epidemiology *147*
  examination at six to eight weeks
    228
  high–frequency 82
  impedance measurement 157, 161

incremental yield of screening 156
intervention 149–58
litigation 219
meningitis 157–8
neonatal examination 226
parental awareness 158
parental observations 154
research requirements 161–2
risk factors *147*
school entry sweep test 157, 159
screening 87, 146–62, 150–1
  evaluation 162
  intermediate 156–7, 158–9
  neonatal *147*, 151–4, 152–3, 160,
    161
  prerequisites 154
sensorineural 146, *147*
  congenital 78, 149
  measures 161–2
  with middle-ear disease 155
  progressive 151
staff training 218
testing between 18–42 months
  156–7
unilateral 149
heart disease, congenital 4, 82, 96–100
early detection 96–7
identification 97–8
physical examination 105
referral 99–100
routine examination 98
surveillance programme examination
  228, 229
symptoms 105
heart murmurs 97, 99, 105, 226
height 115
charts 119, 121
  velocity 119
monitoring 114–15
height measurement
after school entry 123
examination at 3¼–3½ years 231
examination at eighteen to
  twenty-four months 230
examination at five years 232
frequency 122–3
parental height 121

referral 123
techniques 117, 119
hepatitis 43
hepatitis B vaccine 42, 57, 217
hernia 102, 107
hip
acquired disorders 96
defects 218
extension in neonate 117
instability management 93–4
limited abduction 94, 104
screening test 3, 4
hip, congenital dislocation 4, 82, 85,
  92–6
causes 92
defined 92
early detection 93
incidence 92–3
instability management 93–4
neonatal examination 96, 226
physical examination 103–4
risk factors 94, 103
screening
  monitoring 104
  policy 95–6
  tests 94–5
  universal 93
ultrasound scanning 95, 104
HIV infection, anonymized testing
  132
homeless family accommodation 12
Homestart 26, 72
home visiting 21, 216–17
programmes 71
homocystinuria 132
hospital staff 20
housing needs 11–12
hydrocephalus 125
hydrocoele 102, 107
hyperbilirubinaemia, conjugated 138
hypercholesterolaemia, familial 135,
  138
hypertension 100–1
physical examination 105–6
hypertrophic obstructive
  cardiomyopathy 98
hypospadias 102

hypothyroidism 6, 85, 115
    biochemical 132
    congenital 130–1
    Down's syndrome 131
    early detection 78
    growth monitoring 111
    juvenile–onset 121
    screening 137, 181
    testing 22, 214, 217, 218
        neonatal examination 226
    weight gain 112

immunization 18, 217
    litigation 219
    rates 57
    uptake increase 41–2
impairment, terminology 15
impedance measurement 157, 161
infectious disease
    incidence reduction 41–4
    prevention 217
information
    ethical considerations 27–8
    sheets 25
    systems 7, 217
injury prevention 220
injury, unintentional 45–7, 48–9, 50
    intervention programmes 47
    misconceptions 47
    monitoring 50
    mortality 46
    multi-agency planning 50
    prevention strategies 46, 47, 48–9,
        50
    risk reduction 58
innovation needs 17
interagency collaboration 213
    health promotion programme 224
intracranial tumour 111
intrauterine growth retardation 115
iron deficiency 6
iron deficiency anaemia 140–5, 230
    behavioural deficit 140–1
    developmental deficit 140–1
    prevalence 141, 144
    primary prevention 142–3, 144

screening 141–2, 144–5
iron supplements 142, 143, 144
    overdose 143

jaundice 228
    benign prolonged 135
    breast-milk 51, 135
juvenile arthritis

Kawasaki disease 105

laboratory tests 130–8
    familial hypercholesterolaemia 135
    haemoglobinopathies 134–5
    liver disease 135
    subclinical lead poisoning 136
    urine infection 133
lactation establishment 51–2
language
    quality 186
    screening instrument 208
    support 192
    therapy 193
    see also speech
language acquisition
    delayed 6, 180, 189, 207
    examination at 3¼–3½ years 231
    expressive 207
    high-prevalence low-severity
        disability 184, *185*, 186–94
    intervention 192–4
    normal 208
        variation 184, , 186
    otitis media with effusion 148
    promotion 65–7
    reading 66, 67
    secondary impairment 186
    slow 189–90
    variation 188
    writing 66
language development
    child abuse 186
    co-morbidity 186
    comprehension deficit 190, 191

delay 186
deprivation 186
  environmental 206
detection of problems 207
home-visiting programme 193
long-term benefits of intervention
    193–4
markers 189
neglect 186
normal 191–2, 208
nursery education 192, 194
outcome for delayed 187–8
severe difficulties 208
support 208
language impairment 6
  correlates *187*
  disability
  environmental deprivation 194
  family's mother tongue 191
  prognosis 190
  reading 190, 196
  referral 191
  secondary 188–94
    defined 188–9
  specific 187
  staff training 218
lay workers 26
lead intoxication, subclinical 136, 138
learning, critical period 150
learning difficulties, severe 180
learning disability
  borderline/mild 195
  global 206–7
    mild 184
  specific 184, 195–6
length monitoring 114–15
  measurement techniques 117
life-threatening event *57*
linkworker schemes 25
listeriosis 43
literacy 25
litigation 7, 218
  missed diagnoses 131
liver disease 135
  screening 138
local radio programmes 25
loneliness 64–5

low birth weight babies 71–2
  iron deficiency anaemia 140, 144
  length measurement 122
  retinopathy of prematurity 174
  support for mother 181

McCormick Toy Test 156
maple syrup urine disease 132
Marfan's syndrome 97
maternal and child health nurse 21
media and immunization uptake 41
medical examination, school entrant
    103, 232
medicines, sugar-based *55*, *56*
medium-chain acylCoA deficiency 132
meningitis *147*, 157–8
meningococcal disease 42, 43
mental handicap, *see* learning
    difficulties, severe
mental health 7
  mother 63–5
  parent concerns 33
metabolic disorders, inherited 132
microcephaly 125–6
middle ear disease 155
  see also otitis media with effusion
midwives 20, 225–6
milk
  iron-fortified formula 143, 144
  unmodified cow's 143, 144
MMR vaccine 229
monitoring of service 18
mood disorder 36
  mothers 63
motor delay 195
multi-agency planning 214, 217
muscular dystrophy 133
  screening 137
  see also Duchenne muscular
      dystrophy
myopia 166, 171

near vision 169
neglect 33
  language development 186

246 Health for all children

neglect (*cont.*)
  prevention 68–70
  risk 22
  weight gain 113
neonatal examination 4, 225–6
  early detection 79–80
  eyes 174
  hearing tests 5
  physical 103
network
  social 26, 64–5
  support 24
neuroblastoma 136, 138
neurodevelopmental problems 174
Newpin 26, 72–3
nine-centile chart 116, , 122
non-accidental injury 218
Noonan's syndrome 111
  growth charts 123
nursery education 192
  language development 194
nutrition 51–4
  education in iron deficiency 143
  health information 52–3
  national guidelines 58
  parental support/advice 3
  specialist advice 53–4

obesity 113–14
optometrists 177
oral disease 54–7
orthoptic examination 168
orthoptic service, community 6
Ortolani–Barlow manoeuvre 94
osteogenesis imperfecta *181*
otitis media with effusion 146–9,
    156–7
  management 157
  monitoring 159
  persistence
  quality of life 161
  referral 157
  treatment 149

paediatricians 20

palatal dysfunction 194
paraprofessionals 26
parental responsibility 19
parenthood
  education for 62–3
  preparation 62–3, 181
parenting
  difficulties 72–3
  good enough skills 61–3
parents
  advice 3
  child neglect/abuse 33
  children with special needs 57
  communication of severe disabilities
      183
  education 31
  failure to recognize defects 81–2
  growth monitoring value 110
  health promotion programme 216,
      218
  hearing loss awareness 158
  height 121
  listening to 23
  mental health 198
  professional advice 36, 81–2
  role in early detection 80
  smoking reduction 44–5
  speech intervention programmes 194
  support 3
    projects 72–3
  teenage 32
  under stress 57
patent ductus arteriosus 97
peer review 17
periodontal disease 54, 55
personal child health records 7, 217,
      219–21
  duplicates 221
  health promotion programme 225
  ownership 221
  school use 221
  translations for ethnic minorities 221
personal strategies 13
phenylketonuria 6, 130–2
  early detection 78
  neonatal examination 226
  screening 137, 181

testing 214, 217, 218, 220
phonological awareness 67
physical examination 4
  8-week 90–1
  asthma 101–2, 106
  at 3¼–3½ years 231
  congenital heart disease 96–100
  eyes 174
  genitalia abnormalities 102
  hypertension 100–1, 105–6
  individual procedures 92–102
  neonatal 90–1, 103, 226
  school entrant 91–2
  two months 91
picture tests 169
pneumococcal infection 134
Portage home teaching scheme 73
postnatal depression 63
poverty 11, 31
  industrialized countries 32
  psychological problems 198–9
precocious puberty 115
pregnancy 43
  smoking 45
prematurity 80
  correction for 182
  iron deficiency anaemia 140
  iron supplementation 144
  patent ductus arteriosus 97
pre-school age group 1
preventive model of health promotion
    11
primary health care team 1–2
  defined 16
  examination of child 227, 228, 229,
      230, 231
  health promotion responsibility 20
  population perspective 16
  resource targeting 3
primary prevention 1
  asthma 101–2
  behavioural problems 67–8
  care of next infant 57
  congenital heart disease 100
  dental disease 56–7
  health promotion programme
      222–3

infectious disease incidence reduction
    41–4
  low-prevalence high-severity
      disabilities 180–1
  nutrition 51–4
  opportunities 41–58
  psychological problems 67–8
pseudobulbar palsy 181
psychological problems 67–8, 184
  identification 198
  incidence 197
  intervention 198–9
  mild 196–9
  persistence 197
  poverty 198–9
  service provision 199
  social deprivation 198–9
psychometrics 202
psychosocial problems 179
puberty
  constitutional delay 115
  precocious 115
public health 16
  growth monitoring 110
  responsibilities , 18
  staff 20
puerperal psychosis, acute 63

quality of life
  early detection 78
  otitis media with effusion 161

radiological screening tests 131–8
  atlanto–axial instability 136
reading 66, 67
  difficulties 175
  dyslexia 173–4
  language development 196
    delay 190
  problems 195
  speech delay 190
referral
  criteria 170
  disability 207
  health promotion programme 223

referral (*cont.*)
indications 231
language impairment 191
pathways 3–4
screening programmes 88–9
refractive error 166, 167
family history 171
refugees 91
research 2
health promotion 37
resources
implications 2
targeting 3
retinoblastoma 164
retinopathy of prematurity 164, 174,
219
rubella
sensorineural hearing loss 151
vaccination 181
Russell–Silver syndrome 111

school
children requiring support 203–4
entrant medical examination 103,
232
health issues 203
health service 232
nurse 91, 232
special needs education 78–9, 231
scotopic sensitivity syndrome 173
screening 82–9, 224
anxiety 85
attitudes 84–6
criteria for programmes/tests 83–4
cystic fibrosis 137
defined 82–3
evaluation of tests 86–7, 88
formal 84
hypothyroidism 131, 137
incremental yield 84, 86–7
information provision 86
iron deficiency anaemia 141–2,
144–5
litigation 85–6
liver disease 138
muscular dystrophy 137

opportunist 84
phenylketonuria 131, 137
potential harm 85
secondary disease prevention 14
validity 201
screening programmes
biochemical 6
contracts 18
developmental 6
formal 82
hearing 5
iron deficiency 6
management 87–9
missed conditions 7
monitoring 88
referral 3–4, 88–9
review 4
standards 214
vision 5–6
Wilson and Jungner criteria 83,
86–7, 199–200
secondary prevention 77–9
formal screening programmes 82
self-empowerment model of health
promotion 11
service provision, coordinated 10
sexual abuse 70
Sheridan Gardiner cards 169
Shigella diarrhoea 43
short stature 115
idiopathic 111
sickle cell disease 25, 134
signing 150
Silver–Russell syndrome 115
skeletal dysplasia 115
skin creases, asymmetric 94–5
smoking
asthma 101, 106
Health of the Nation target 44
otitis media with effusion risk 147
passive 44, 45, 101
primary prevention 45
reduction 44
Snellen letter chart 166, 169, 171, 232
social class, health outcomes 11
social deprivation 198–9
social network 24, 26, 64–5

social services 70
social skills 33
social support 23–5
social worth 23
somatizers 68
Sonksen–Silver test 169
special needs 11, 57, 231
  education 78–9, 231
  Portage home teaching scheme 73
speech
  acquisition 65
  delayed 6, 180
    reading 190
  discrimination tasks 156–7
  high-prevalence low-severity
    disability 184, 185, 186–94
  therapy 193
  see also language
speech impairment
  cleft palate 194
  disability *181*
  palatal dysfunction 194
  staff training 218
spina bifida occulta 85
splenic sequestration crises 134
squint 165, 166, 167, 229, 231
  detection 171, 172
stammering 194
stress 11
  coping ability 24
  factors 22
  parent support 57
  somatizers 68
Stycar test 169
subdural effusion 125
sudden infant death syndrome 29, 218
  incidence 44
  mental health of mother 63
  prevention 44
  risk *43*
    reduction 58, 226
  weight gain 113
sudden unexpected death in infancy 44
sugar 55
support 23–5
  intensive service 72–4
surveillance 1, 2, 9, 14, 17–18

antenatal 181
contracts 18
Core Programme 36
health promotion 27
non-specific oversight 14
preconceptional 181
preschool 91
service 14
surveillance programme
  core 225–32
  eighteen to twenty-four months
    229–30
  first two weeks 226–7
  five years 232
  neonatal examination 225–6
  records 225
  six to eight weeks 227–8
  six to nine months 229
  three and a quarter to three and a
    half years 230–2
  two, three and four months 228–9
  weighing 228–9
sweep test 232

tall stature 111
teenage parents 32
teeth
  brushing 55, 56
  traumatic damage 56
telephone service 36
testes
  descent 4
  examination at 3¼–3½ years
    231
  undescended 102, 106–7, 228
thalassaemia 134
  iron deficiency 143, 144
thyroid-stimulating hormone 131
thyrotoxicosis 115
toxocariasis 43
toxoplasmosis 43
translation services 25
trusts 213
tuberculosis
  control strategy 57
  prevention 42, 217

tuberculosis (*cont.*)
  screening 91
Turner's syndrome 115, 121
  growth charts 123
  growth monitoring 111
  otitis media with effusion 147

ultrasound scanning for hip dislocation
      95, 104
undernutrition 112
urinary tract infection 133
  diagnosis 137
urine infection 133
uveitis 164

vaccine
  damage 41
  new 42
vegetarians/vegans 53
ventricular septal defects 97
vesico–ureteric reflux 133
vision
  examination at 3¼–3½ years 231
  examination at five years 232
  parental concerns 230
  screening 5–6
vision assessment
  cooperation 169–70
  coverage 169–70
  near vision 169
  orthoptic examination 168
  preschool child 168–9
  referral criteria 170
  visual acuity measurement 168
vision defects 165–77
  colour vision 173, 175–6, 177
  dyslexia 173–4
  family disorders 174
  non-disabling 175
  non-incapacitating 165–70
  screening 5–6
    community 171–3
    preschool 170

school entrant 171
  secondary 172
  staff training 218
vision impairment
  disabling 165–6
  early detection 164–5
  secondary disability 165
visual acuity 166
  assessment at school entry 172–3
  disability 170
  distance vision 169
  impaired 166
  measurement 168
  school entry testing 175
  Sonksen–Silver test 169
  testing 176
visual failure, progressive 165
vitamin K 51, 52
  deficiency 135
  litigation 219
  prophylaxis 53
voluntary organizations 26

walking
  age 195
  see also gait
weight
  distance charts 127
  measurement techniques 117
  velocity reference 127
weight monitoring 112–14
  centile shifts 114
  overweight baby 113–14
  regression to the mean 113
  slow gain 112–13
whole body irradiation 111
Wilson and Jungner criteria for
      screening programmes 83, 86–7,
      199–200
workload 2
writing 66

zinc protoporphyrin 140